Surgical Techniques in Sports Medicine

Elbow Surgery

Surgical Techniques in Sports Medicine

Elbow Surgery

François M Kelberine MD

Professor of Orthopaedic Surgery
Polyclinique du Parc Rambot
Aix-en-Provence, France

Wasim Khan, MRCS, PhD, FRCS(Tr&Orth)

Post CCT Fellow
Cardiff and Vale Orthopaedic Centre
Cardiff, UK

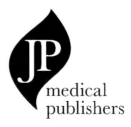

JP
medical
publishers

London • Philadelphia • Panama City • New Delhi

© 2016 JP Medical Ltd.
Published by JP Medical Ltd
83 Victoria Street, London, SW1H 0HW, UK
Tel: +44 (0)20 3170 8910
Fax: +44 (0)20 3008 6180
Email: info@jpmedpub.com
Web: www.jpmedpub.com

ISBN: 978-1-909836-39-6

British Library Cataloguing in Publication Data
A catalogue record for this book is available from the British Library

Library of Congress Cataloging in Publication Data
A catalog record for this book is available from the Library of Congress

Commissioning Editor:	Steffan Clements
Development Editor:	Gavin Smith
Design:	Designers Collective Ltd

Foreword

Education is one of the key missions of EFOST, the European Federation of National Associations of Orthopaedic Sport Traumatology. The *Surgical Techniques in Sports Medicine* series is the educational flagship of EFOST, and provides an invaluable supplement to the experience afforded by the international EFOST Travelling Fellowship.

This series of highly illustrated handbooks, each dedicated to a specific anatomical region, is aimed at established surgeons, fellows in orthopaedic sports traumatology and residents in orthopaedics. It comprises much more than the simple scientific evidence behind each procedure. The aim instead is to impart practical knowledge arising from the direct experience of highly experienced surgeons, who describe reliable surgical procedures in a practical, easy-to-follow manner that will be of great value to orthopaedic and sports trauma surgeons alike.

Surgical Techniques in Sports Medicine is the fruit of five years' work by the three immediate past presidents of EFOST and is testament to how far EFOST has come since its foundation in 1992.

We hope that you find this book, and the others in the series, a useful resource.

Gernot Felmet
President, EFOST
Francois Kelberine
Series Editor
Wasim Khan
Editor

October 2015

Contents

Contributors

Elie Choufani, MD
Department of Paediatric Orthopaedics
Timone Children's Hospital
Aix Marseille University
Marseille, France

Emilio Delli Sante, MD
Orthopaedic–Traumatology Department
New Sassuolo Hospital
Sassuolo, Italy

Felice Di Palma, MD
Orthopaedic–Traumatology Department
New Sassuolo Hospital
Sassuolo, Italy

Konstantinos T. Ditsios, MD, PhD
Assistant Professor, Department of Orthopaedics
Aristotle University of Thessaloniki
Thessaloniki, Greece

Nikolaos A Doxariotis, MD
Orthopaedic Surgeon
Department of Orthopaedics
University of Thessalia
Larissa, Greece

Denise Eygendaal, MD, PhD
Professor of Orthopaedic Surgery
Amphia Hospital
Breda, The Netherlands

Michael Hantes, MD, PhD
Associate Professor of Orthopaedics
Department of Orthopaedic Surgery
University of Thessalia
Larissa, Greece

Neil E Jarvis, MB, ChB, FRCS (Tr&Orth)
Sports and Upper Extremity Fellow
SPM Orthopaedics
AZ Monica
Antwerp, Belgium

Jean-Luc Jouve, MD
Professor of Paediatric Orthopaedic Surgery
Department of Paediatric Orthopaedics
Timone Children's Hospital
Aix Marseille University
Marseille, France

Polykarpos I Kiorpelidis, MD
Orthopaedic Surgeon
Department of Orthopaedic Surgery
University of Thessalia
Larissa, Greece

Izaäk F Kodde, MD
Orthopaedic Surgeon
Department of Orthopaedic Surgery,
Upper Limb Unit
Amphia Hospital
Breda, The Netherlands

Franck Launay, MD
Professor of Paediatric Orthopaedic Surgery
Department of Paediatric Orthopaedics
Timone Children's Hospital
Aix Marseille University
Marseille, France

Gürsel Leblebicioğlu, MD
Professor of Orthopaedic Surgery and Traumatology
European Diploma of Hand Surgery FESSH
Division of Hand Surgery
Department of Orthopaedic Surgery and Traumatology
Hacettepe University, Faculty of Medicine
Ankara, Turkey

Pierre Mansat, MD, PhD
Professor of Orthopaedic Surgery
Department of Orthopaedics and Traumatology
Chief of Upper Limb Unit
Toulouse University
Pierre-Paul Riquet Hospital
Toulouse, France

Mahmut Nedim Doral, MD
Professor of Orthopaedic Surgery
Department of Orthopaedic Surgery and Traumatology
Department of Sports Medicine
Hacettepe University
Ankara, Turkey

Fabio Nicoletta, MD
Orthopaedic–Traumatology Department
New Sassuolo Hospital
Sassuolo, Italy

Luigi A Pederzini, MD
Professor of Orthopaedic Surgery
Orthopaedic–Traumatology Department
New Sassuolo Hospital
Sassuolo, Italy

Sébastien Pesenti, MD
Department of Paediatric Orthopaedics
Timone Children's Hospital
Aix Marseille University
Marseille, France

Seval Tanrıkulu, MD
Orthopaedic Surgeon
Department of Orthopaedics and Traumatology
Hand Surgeon, Department of Hand Surgery
Ankara Numune Training and Research Hospital
Ankara, Turkey

Emanuele Tripoli, MD
Orthopaedic–Traumatology Department
New Sassuolo Hospital
Sassuolo, Italy

Robert G Turner, MC Bch, FRCS
Consultant Trauma and Orthopaedic Surgeon
Princess Royal Hospital, Telford
Royal Shrewsbury Hospital, Shrewsbury
Keele University Medical School
Stoke-on-Trent, UK

Akin Üzümcügil, MD
Asssistant Professor of Orthopaedic Surgery
Department of Hand Surgery
Hacettepe University
Ankara, Turkey

Roger van Riet, MD, PhD
Orthopaedic Elbow Surgeon
Department of Orthopaedic Surgery and Traumatology
AZ Monica
Antwerp, Belgium

Melanie Vandenberghe, MD
Senior Orthopaedic Registrar
Department of Orthopaedic Surgery and Traumatology
AZ Monica
Antwerp, Belgium

Sokratis E Varitimidis, MD
Associate Professor of Orthopaedics
University of Thessalia
Larissa, Greece

Elke Viehweger, MD, PhD
Professor of Paediatric Orthopaedic Surgery
Department of Paediatric Orthopaedics
Timone Children's Hospital
Aix Marseille University
Marseille, France

Adam Watts, MBBS, BSc, FRCS(Tr & Ortho)
Consultant Upper Limb Surgeon
Upper Limb Unit, Wrightington Hospital
Visiting Professor, Department of Materials
University of Manchester
Manchester, UK

W Jaap Willems, MD, PhD
Shoulder Unit
Lairesse Kliniek
Amsterdam, The Netherlands

1 Arthroscopic debridement for osteochondritis dissecans of the capitellum

Indications

- The natural history varies and while some lesions heal spontaneously, other detach. Unstable fragments generally benefit from fixation
- Once a semi-detached or completely detached loose body is formed, fixation is generally not possible and debridement will be necessary, with simultaneous treatment of the defect with microfracture or autologous osteochondral graft transplantation, often from the knee
- Stable fragments with open growth plates generally do not require any surgery

Preoperative assessment

Clinical assessment

- This rare condition of childhood and adolescence is more common in high-level athletes involved in elbow overuse activities, e.g. baseball or gymnastics
- The patients describe pain and often some loss of flexion and extension. Locking suggests a loose body
- On examination, the range of motion is compared with the contralateral side to demonstrate any loss of movement
- Effusion is best demonstrated in the posterolateral soft spot
- The elbow is also examined for stability, and although gymnasts are generally hyperlax, ligamentous instability is rarely present

Imaging assessment

Radiographs

- Anteroposterior and lateral radiographs of the elbow, supplemented with an anteroposterior radiograph with the elbow in 45° of flexion, generally reveal the lesion (**Figure 1.1**), but do not give any information regarding the stability of the fragment

Computed tomography (CT)

- CT with three-dimensional imaging is better at determining the location and size of the lesion (**Figure 1.2**)

Magnetic resonance imaging (MRI)

- MRI findings correlate well with the International Cartilage Repair Society staging

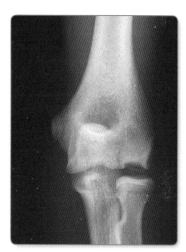

Figure 1.1
Radiograph of the left elbow of a young gymnast showing a small loose bone fragment representing an unstable osteochondritis dissecans lesion.

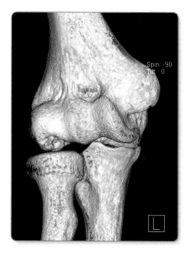

Figure 1.2
Three-dimensional CT of the same patient as shown in Figure 1.1.

and give information on the degree of stability of the lesion, enabling optimal treatment planning (**Figure 1.3**)

Timing for surgery

- Surgery is performed when pain and loss of movement persist and MRI suggests instability. In the rare event of the elbow being locked, more urgent surgery is indicated

Surgical preparation

Surgical equipment

- It is preferable to perform the procedure arthroscopically. A standard arthroscopic setup consists of a camera system, pump, and a shaver. Pump pressure is generally lower than in other larger joints, and 30–40 mmHg is usually sufficient. Gravity-assisted flow with suspended normal saline bags can be used instead of a pump, with the pressure controlled by the distance between the patient and the fluid bags
- Either a small 2.7 mm or a large 4.5 mm diameter arthroscope is needed depending on the age and size of the patient. In smaller children a small arthroscope is preferable
- Smaller 3.5 mm shaver blades and burrs are mandatory, especially when working in the posterolateral compartment
- Radiofrequency is rarely needed
- Instruments for microfracture are helpful, but Kirschner wires can be used instead

Equipment positioning

- While the patient is mostly positioned in lateral decubitus or prone position, the arthroscopic tower is placed at the other side of the table
- The instruments as well as the nurse are positioned next to the surgeon; the instruments can also be put on a small instrument table, placed over the patient

Patient positioning

- After general anesthesia, preferably with an interscalene block, the patient is positioned either in the lateral decubitus or prone position
- A tourniquet around the upper arm is used to allow better intra-articular visualization. The tourniquet pressure should not exceed 100 mmHg above the systolic blood pressure. Tourniquet time should not exceed 2 hours
- The upper arm is positioned in an arm holder with the elbow freely mobile (**Figure 1.4**). It is important to ensure that the elbow can be maximally flexed intraoperatively to allow a greater exposure of the capitellum
- Some surgeons prefer the supine position with traction at the hand, and the elbow suspended in 90° of flexion. The disadvantage of this position is that the elbow is not as freely mobile as in the earlier position
- During positioning, care should be taken to prevent pressure on nerves including the peroneal nerve, and ulnar nerve. Pressure on the lateral cutaneous nerve of the thigh should be avoided in the lateral decubitus position. In the

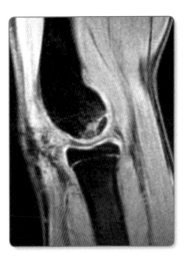

Figure 1.3 MRI showing osteochondritis dissecans lesion with intact overlying cartilage.

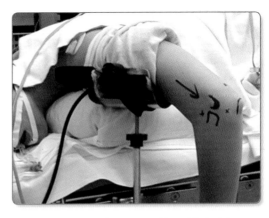

Figure 1.4 Patient in the prone position with the left upper arm in a support.

prone position, the chest and abdomen should be free, and this is achieved with cylindrical pillows under the shoulders and pelvis. Extreme abduction of the arm should be avoided to prevent stretching of the brachial plexus

Further preparation

- When working in the prone position, it is important to orient the lateral and medial sides
- The author recommends marking the anatomic landmarks, portal sites, and course of the ulnar nerve (**Figures 1.5** and **1.6**)
- The elbow and forearm are draped after preparing the skin in a standard fashion

Surgical technique

Portals and joint inspection

- Normal saline is injected through the distal posterolateral portal in the soft area. The elbow

extends when enough pressure inside the joint is achieved (**Figure 1.7**). The safest entry for the arthroscope is through the proximal medial portal, ventrally from the intermuscular septum (**Figure 1.6**). A thorough inspection of the ventral joint area is performed
- An anterolateral portal (**Figure 1.5**) is made from outside in after checking the direction with a needle. This portal should be at the level of the joint line, enabling instruments to enter the ventral area of the radiocapitellar joint
- With the elbow flexed, the lesion is mostly visible as it is generally situated more dorsally on the capitellum
- Loose bodies in the ventral joint area can be removed. The scope is then inserted posterolaterally through the soft spot. Alternatively, when using a larger scope with less space in the soft area, a more distal ulnar portal can be used for the scope

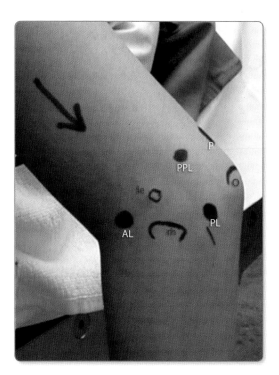

Figure 1.5 View from the lateral side of the left elbow with portals and landmarks outlined. AL, anterolateral portal; le, lateral epicondyle; o, olecranon; rh, radial head; PL, posterolateral portal; PPL, proximal posterolateral portal; P, posterior portal through triceps tendon.

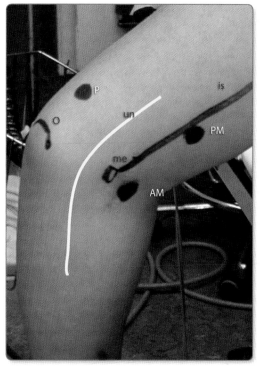

Figure 1.6 View from the medial side of the elbow with portals and landmarks outlined. AM, anteromedial portal; is, intermuscular septum; me, medial epicondyle; o, olecranon; PM, proximo medial portal; P, posterior portal through triceps; un, ulnar nerve.

- A second portal is created 3–5 mm laterally to insert a shaver or other instruments (**Figure 1.8**)
- After removal of synovial tissue in case of local synovitis, the capitellum lesion can be visualized adequately
- Through this portal, the dorsal part of the proximal radioulnar joint can be inspected as well as the ulnohumeral joint:

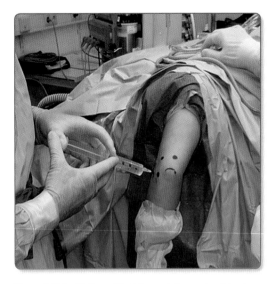

Figure 1.7 Instillation of fluid through the posterolateral portal in the soft spot to distend the joint.

- While carefully extending the elbow, the ulnohumeral joint line can be followed till the olecranon fossa is visualized
- Under direct vision, a posterior portal through the triceps tendon can be made. The scope can be inserted through this portal and the whole dorsal joint inspected, starting medially in the ulnar gutter looking for loose bodies, turning laterally along lateral the border of the capitellum and the radial head
- The scope can be inserted through the portal through the triceps. The whole dorsal compartment can be inspected, looking out for the olecranon tip for orientation. Firstly the olecranon fossa is inspected. Then the scope is turned medially, looking into the ulnar gutter: sometimes loose bodies are hidden in this medial part. Returning to the olecranon tip, the scope is directed laterally, looking into the lateral gutter; proceeding distally (which is sometimes difficult with the scope through the triceps portal and easier through the proximal posterolateral portal) one can visualise the radial head and posterior aspect of the capitellum
- A more lateral portal, the proximal posterolateral portal, can be made if needed just next to the triceps tendon to facilitate surgery or removing loose bodies from the posterior joint compartment

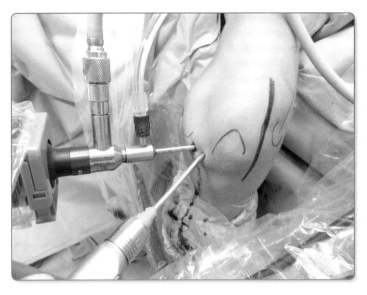

Figure 1.8 Arthroscopy through two portals in the posterolateral soft spot with small joint instruments.

Procedure

- After the general inspection of the elbow, surgery is performed through the two appropriate portals
- If the fragment is still in place, its stability is assessed with a probe
- If the fragment is stable, drilling is performed either anterograde through the cartilage with a thin Kirschner wire, or retrograde from outside using an aiming device similar to one used for anterior cruciate ligament reconstruction. Drilling into the demarcated sclerotic area between the lesion and the healthy capitellum enhances vascular ingrowth
- An unstable semi-detached lesion (**Figure 1.9**) can be fixed with or without bone grafting the bed of the lesion. This is generally performed through an open approach, preferably using biodegradable pins for fixation
- For a detached lesion, the rim of the cartilage is abraded, and the subchondral plate is drilled with a burr or microfractured with an awl or pick (**Figure 1.10**). Alternatively, a Kirschner wire inserted through the distal ulnar portal can be used (**Figure 1.11**). Flexing the elbow maximally allows the entire area to be treated (**Figure 1.12**)

Possible perioperative complications

- General complications are related to the anesthesia or patient positioning

- Local complications include vascular and neurologic complications
- The brachial artery is potentially at risk, although it is protected by the brachial muscle when it is running ventral to the muscle
- Dorsally the ulnar nerve runs just outside the ulnar gutter of the joint, and medial portal

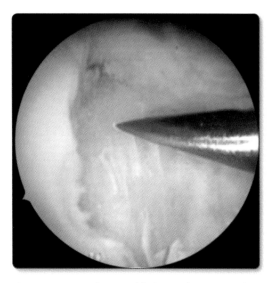

Figure 1.10 Micro-fracture of the lesion after removal of the loose fragments.

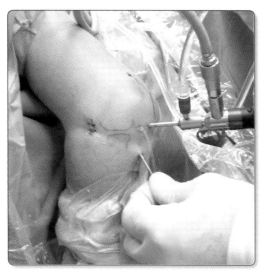

Figure 1.11 Scoping through one of the posterolateral portals and inserting the Kirschner wire through the distal ulnar portal.

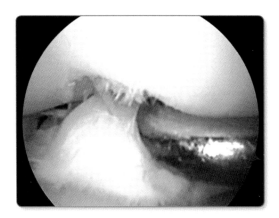

Figure 1.9 Unstable semi-detached fragment.

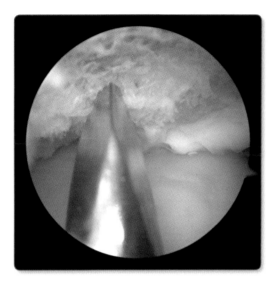

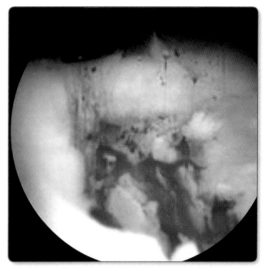

Figure 1.12 Same patient as shown in Figure 1.11 with the Kirschner wire on the defect.

Figure 1.13 Bleeding from after the microfracture site after deflation of the tourniquet.

placement should be accurate to avoid injury to the nerve. Marking the course of the nerve preoperatively helps avoid injury to the nerve
- The deep branch of the radial nerve, which has mainly motor fibers, runs ventrally close to the capsule at the level of the center of the radial head. The superficial branch with its mainly sensory fibers runs more ventrally and should be avoided when making the anterolateral portal. Blunt dissection with an artery forcep before inserting the scope, and directing the scope obliquely rather than parallel to the joint line, help avoid injury to the nerve

Closure

- On completion of the procedure, the tourniquet is deflated and bleeding from the bone bed visualized (**Figure 1.13**)

Further reading

Satake H, Takahara M, Harada M, Maruyama M. Pre-operative imaging criteria for unstable osteochondritis dissecans of the capitellum. Clin Orthop Relat Res 2013; 471:1137–1143.

Takahara M, Mura N, Sasaki J, et al. Classification, treatment and outcome of osteochondritis dissecans

- The joint is in close proximity to the skin, and the portals should be closed. A standard pressure bandage is applied
- A broad arm sling is used for 1 week

Postoperative management

- Active and passive exercises, as well as isometric exercises of the upper arm muscles, can be started at 1 week postoperatively

Outpatient follow-up

- MRI performed at 4 months should visualize a new fibrocartilaginous layer. At this stage, the young athlete is allowed to recommence sporting activities

of the humeral capitellum. J Bone Joint Surg Am 2007; 89:1205–1214.

van den Ende KI, Mcintosh AL, Adams JE, Steinmann SP. Osteochondritis dissecans of the capitellum: a review of the literature and a distal ulnar portal. Arthroscopy 2011; 27:122–128.

2 Arthroscopic treatment of osteochondritis dissecans using mosaicplasty

Indications

- The treatment of osteochondritis dissecans (OCD) is based on the separation of the osteochondral fragment
- Stable early lesions are managed nonoperatively, and avoidance of sports and repetitive stress on the elbow is usually sufficient to allow complete healing of the lesion
- Surgery is the treatment of choice for unstable lesions, loose bodies, and symptomatic lesions that fail nonoperative treatment after a period of 3–6 months

Preoperative assessment

Clinical assessment

- OCD typically affects the young adolescent athlete from 13 to 16 years of age involved in high-demand, repetitive overhead throwing or weight-bearing activities, e.g. baseball, gymnastics, racquet sports, American football, and weight lifting
- OCD can cause recurrent pain, progressive dysfunction, and limited range of motion. The patient may also complain of popping and clicking. The young athletes will complain of pain and limitation of activities affecting their ability to participate in sport
- On examination there may be secondary joint contracture and joint swelling

Imaging assessment

- Although lesions have been reported in the trochlea, radial head, and olecranon, the most common site of OCD of the elbow is the capitellum
- Panner's disease is a differential diagnosis and should not be confused with true OCD;

Panner's disease is most common from 4 to 8 years of age and involves the entire ossification center, not only the anterolateral capitellum

Radiographs

- In the early stage, radiographs may be normal or only show localized radiolucencies or bone rarefactions
- In the advanced stage, loose intra-articular bodies and joint irregularities may be seen

Magnetic resonance imaging (MRI)

- MRI has become the standard imaging modality for OCD and provides an accurate assessment of the size, extent, and stability of the lesion
- Determination of lesion stability and the integrity of the articular cartilage cap is important in deciding between nonoperative and operative treatment

Surgical preparation

Surgical equipment

- Arthroscopy stack and intruments including a 4.5 mm 30° arthroscope

Equipment positioning

- The surgeon stands with the operating table at chest level to prevent contamination of the dependent hand. An arm board is placed parallel to the operating table at the level of the arm
- All equipment is mounted on a portable rolling platform
- The monitor, digital recorder, light and camera control and pump with irrigation bags are placed on the opposite side of the patient
- A mayo tray is on the right of the surgeon
- An assistant is on the left of the surgeon

Patient positioning

- The patient is placed in the lateral decubitus position with the shoulder abducted to 90° and the elbow flexed to 90° with the arm in an arm holder secured to the operating table (**Figure 2.1**)
- The ipsilateral hip is externally rotated with the knee exposed to harvest the donor osteochondral tissue for mosaicplasty from the lateral trochlea
- The anesthetist identifies the nerve trunks with electrostimulation and places a catheter before general anesthesia. At the end of the surgical procedure, after an accurate neurovascular examination to exclude neurovascular lesions, a peripheral block is performed for pain relief

Surgical technique

- An examination under anesthesia is performed to assess the range of movement and ligamentous stability
- A tourniquet is applied, and after preparation of the skin with antiseptic solution and draping, the tourniquet is inflated to 250 mmHg
- The elbow joint landmarks, including the medial and lateral epicondyle, ulnar nerve, radial head, and posterior soft spot, are outlined with a skin marker. The soft spot posterolateral portals, supero-anteromedial and supero-anterolateral portals are also marked

- An 18-gauge needle is inserted into the elbow through the 'soft-spot' in the center of the triangle formed by the lateral epicondyle, the radial head, and the olecranon. The joint is distended by injecting 20 mL of normal saline, and a skin incision is made followed by blunt dissection through the soft tissues using an artery clip. The joint is distended by injecting 20 mL of normal saline that shifts the anterior neurovascular structures away. An incision is made in the skin followed by blunt dissection through the soft tissues using an artery clip. A trocar is introduced into this posterolateral portal
- Five portals, three posterior and two anterior, are always used with the skin incision, followed by blunt soft tissue disection
- Posterior compartment arthroscopy is performed first by introducing the arthroscope through the posterolateral portal. Joint distension is achieved by a pump set at 35–50 mmHg. A second portal is established 1.5 cm proximally
- These two portals allow the use of the scope and the shaver at the level of the posterior portion of the radial head and allow a good and complete view of the proximal radioulnar joint. The OCD lesion is identified and prepared to accept the osteochondral cylinder (**Figures 2.2–2.4**)

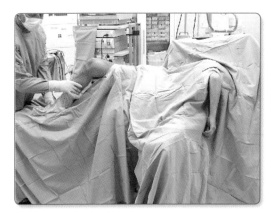

Figure 2.1 Patient positioning in the lateral decubitus position with the elbow exposed, and the hip in external rotation to allow knee arthroscopy for graft harvesting.

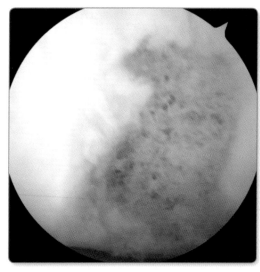

Figure 2.2 Arthroscopic view of osteochondritis dissecans of the capitellum.

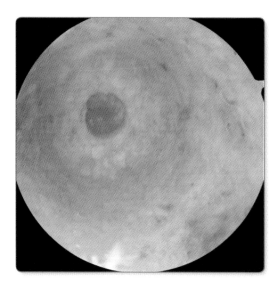

Figure 2.3 Arthroscopic view after drilling the area of osteochondritis dissecans.

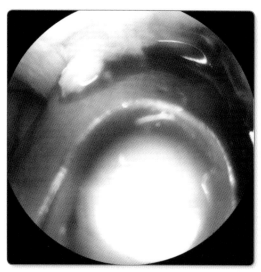

Figure 2.5 Using the mosaicplasty technique, the graft is inserted to restore the normal anatomy.

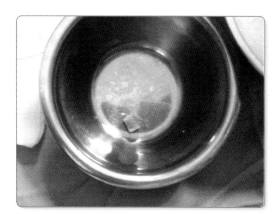

Figure 2.4 Osteochondral cylinder harvested from the lateral femoral trochlea.

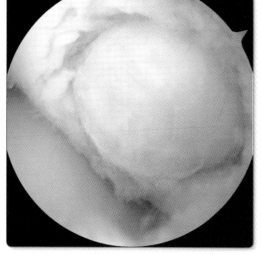

Figure 2.6 The graft is positioned on the lateral humeral condyle to fill the osteochondritis dissecans gap.

- A third posterior portal is placed in the olecranon fossa, close to the medial border of the triceps and oriented 2–3 cm proximal to the olecranon tip
- A mosaicplasty is performed with the oteochondral graft harvested from the lateral femoral trochlea of the contralateral knee arthroscopically

- The 6.5 mm cylindrical osteochondral graft taken from the lateral femoral trochlea is inserted at the prepared recipient site in the elbow lesion. A perpendicular insertion of the cylinder allows a complete coverage of the OCD area. A cylinder press-fit makes the graft stable (**Figures 2.5** and **2.6**)

Possible perioperative complications

- Complications of elbow arthroscopy are the same as for other arthroscopic procedures, including infection, instrument breakage, iatrogenic scuffing of articular surfaces, tourniquet problems, and neurovascular injuries
- Neurological problems are the most commonly reported complications. Most of these are transient injuries

Closure

- After the procedure is completed, range of motion is assessed and the portals are closed in the standard fashion with 3-0 nylon or Prolene sutures
- A sterile compressive dressing is applied
- A long-arm splint is placed posteriorly, to immobilize the arm at 90°

Postoperative management

- Postoperative continuous passive movement commences at day 2, and passive exercises at day 4
- Patients resume normal activity at 4 months postoperatively
- MRI is performed 4 months postoperatively to confirm bone incorporation of the graft

Outpatient follow-up

- After discharge from hospital the patient returns for medication 7 days later
- At 15 days postoperatively all sutures are removed
- The patient has a follow-up appointment every month until new MRI is performed 4 months postoperatively. The patients is then reviewed every year for 2–3 years

Further reading

Baker CL, Romeo AA. Osteochondritis dissecans of the capitellum. Am J Sport Med 2010; 38:1917–1928.

Coates KE, Poehling G. Osteochondritis dissecans lesions and loose bodies of the elbow. In: Pederzini LA,

Bain G, Safran MR (eds), Elbow Arthroscopy. Berlin: Springer-Verlag, 2013: 25–35.

Kandemir U, Fu FH, Mc Mahon P. Elbow injures. Curr Opin Rheumatol 2002; 14:160–167.

Open treatment for lateral epicondylitis

Indications

- Although it is common, lateral epicondylitis is usually self-limiting but can take several weeks or months to resolve. The patient should be counseled and reassured accordingly
- In most cases this condition will resolve within 12 months. Earlier surgery will often be successful, but the surgeon is treating a subsection of patients who would have recovered anyway without surgical treatment
- If conservative treatment has failed, the surgeon should reconsider the differential diagnoses, which include:
  - Posterior interosseus nerve entrapment
  - Posterolateral impingement
  - Posterolateral rotatory instability
  - Lateral synovial fringe or plica
  - Loose bodies
  - Osteochondritis
  - Radiocapitellar arthrosis
  - Cervical radiculopathy
- Surgery should not be performed without an investigation to confirm the diagnosis

Preoperative assessment

Clinical assessment

- The patient is unlikely to have lateral epicondylitis if there is a history of:
  - Dislocation
  - Clicking
  - Locking
  - Instability
  - Stiffness
- The patient should be carefully examined. The patient is unlikely to have lateral epicondylitis if any of the following are noted on examination:
  - Stiffness
  - Distal or posterior tenderness
  - Abnormal neurology

- Tenderness over the common extensor origin suggests lateral epicondylitis pain. Lateral elbow pain on resisted middle finger extension that stresses the extensor carpi radialis brevis (ECRB) tendon is a useful test for lateral epicondylitis
- Tenderness over the radiocapitellar joint or radiocapitellar recess, which lies immediately adjacent, may signify radiocapitellar arthritis or a plica
- Pain on axial compression of the radial forearm with gentle pronation and supination signifies radiocapitellar pathology
- Always assess for posterolateral rotator instability
- Always examine the neck and assess the neurological status

Imaging assessment

Radiographs

- These are usually normal in lateral epicondylitis, but some patients may have a small bone spur in the common extensor area and this should be excised during surgery
- Up to 25% of patients with lateral epicondylitis have calcification within the soft tissue around the lateral epicondyle
- Radiocapitellar arthritis is a differential diagnosis for lateral epicondylitis; if it is present, consider a diagnostic therapeutic injection into the elbow joint

Ultrasonography

- A skilled ultrasonography specialist can identify the changes of lateral epicondylitis
- Typical findings include focal areas of low echogenicity with a background of intrinsic tendinopathy

Magnetic resonance imaging (MRI)

- This will usually show changes of lateral epicondylitis and may also show other pathologies that may be causing the patient's symptoms

Surgical preparation

Surgical equipment

- Standard surgical equipment is used but bone nibbling instruments are useful

Patient positioning

- Supine
- High tourniquet
- Arm resting on arm table

Further preparation

- Up to 20% of patients will have associated intra-articular pathology that may need to be addressed at the same time
- If the surgeon intends to inspect the radiocapitellar joint, use a laminar airflow theatre and give prophylactic antibiotics

Surgical technique

- See **Figure 3.1** for the anatomy. If only performing surgery for lateral epicondylitis, make a 2–3 cm incision centered over the lateral epicondyle (**Figure 3.2**)
- As up to 20% of patients have associated intra-articular pathology, the author recommends inspecting the joint intraoperatively using a slightly longer incision extending distally over the center of the radiocapitellar joint (**Figure 3.3**)
- Identify the aponeurosis between the extensor carpi radialis longus (ECRL) and the extensor digitorum communis (EDC), and incise this to visualize the ECRB tendon underneath. You may need to release some of the ECRL from the lateral supracondylar ridge (**Figure 3.4**)
- Note that the ECRL originates from the lateral humeral supracondylar ridge, from the lateral intermuscular septum, and by a few fibers from the lateral humeral epicondyle. The ECRB and EDC arise from the lateral humeral epicondyle by the common extensor tendon. Proximally, the ECRB lies under the aponeurosis between the EDC and ECRL
- If the tissue planes are not clear, this is most likely to be due to inadequate clearance of the superficial fat and/or fascia
- The pathologic ECRB tissue is removed. This is friable, edematous, greyish, and dull whereas normal tendon is bright, firm, and shiny. Remove any tissue of dubious quality

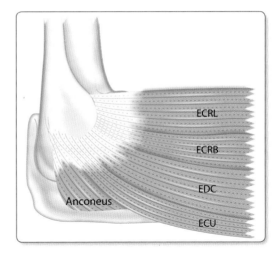

Figure 3.1 Anatomy of the lateral elbow. ECRB, extensor carpi radialis brevis; ECRL, extensor carpi radialis longus; EDC, extensor digitorum communis; ECU, extensor carpi ulnaris.

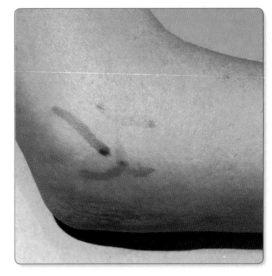

Figure 3.2 Skin incision for tendon surgery: the capitellum and radial head are marked.

- Inspect the undersurface of the EDC in this area. There may be some degenerative tissue present
- Look for calcification or bony prominences. These should also be removed
- The author uses a bone nibbler to decorticate the bone in this area to encourage neovascularization, but some surgeons do

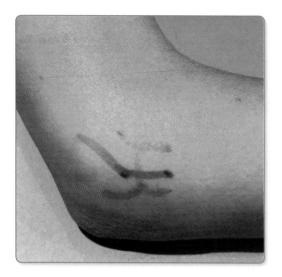

Figure 3.3 Skin incision for tendon surgery and radiocapitellar joint inspection.

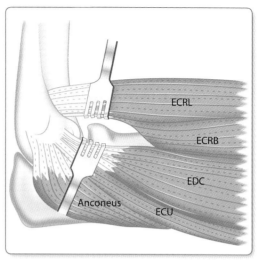

Figure 3.5 Exposure for ECRB debridement and joint inspection. ECRL lifted off EDC to expose ECRB underneath. Distal extension in the same tissue plane to inspect the joint. ECRB, extensor carpi radialis brevis; ECRL, extensor carpi radialis longus; EDC, extensor digitorum communis; ECU, extensor carpi ulnaris.

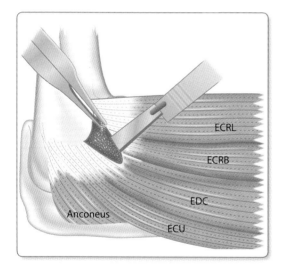

Figure 3.4 Exposure for ECRB debridement. ECRL lifted off EDC to expose ECRB tendon underneath. ECRB, extensor carpi radialis brevis; ECRL, extensor carpi radialis longus; EDC, extensor digitorum communis; ECU, extensor carpi ulnaris.

not do this as it can be a potential source of postoperative pain
- If any intra-articular pathology is suspected, extend the incision between the ECRL and

the EDC to expose the joint. Ensure that the incision does not extend below the midline of the capitellum to avoid injury to the lateral ulnar collateral ligament, which will cause posterolateral instability and lateral elbow pain (**Figure 3.5**)
- If a plica or other pathology is identified, this may be dealt with appropriately
- Elbow stability should be tested before closure to ensure that no iatrogenic injuries have occured

Possible perioperative complications

- Infection
- Stiffness
- Damage to the lateral ulnar collateral ligament, resulting in pain and instability

Closure

- Repair the ECRL to the anterior margin of the EDC aponeurosis using absorbable sutures
- Ensure the knots are buried
- Close the fat layer and skin with absorbable sutures

- Augment wound closure with adhesive Steri-Strips
- Apply a bulky padded dressing, and a sling for comfort

Postoperative management

- Wrist and hand movement is encouraged immediately postoperatively
- Active elbow range of movement exercises commence at 48 hours postoperatively
- Neck and shoulder exercises are encouraged

3 weeks

- Wrist resistance exercises with 1 lb (0.5 kg) weights commenced
- Some patients may benefit from a counterforce elbow brace

6–8 weeks

- Commence heavier activities
- Patient should be advised that maximum recovery can take 4–6 months

Outpatient follow-up

- Two weeks for wound check
- Six weeks to assess progress
- Three-month final review and discharge

Further reading

Nirschl RP, Pettrone FA. Tennis elbow: the surgical treatment of lateral epicondylitis. J Bone Joint Surg Am 1979; 61:832–839.

Jobe FW, Ciccotti MG. Lateral and medial epicondylitis of the elbow. J Am Acad Orthop Surg 1994; 2:1–8.

Faro F, Wolf JM. Lateral epicondylitis: review and current concepts. J Hand Surg Am 2007; 32:1271–1279.

Surgical repair of distal triceps tendon rupture

Indications

The repair of acute (less than 6 weeks) distal triceps ruptures is indicated for:

- Active patients who require sufficient power to maintain the position of the elbow
- All patients unable to maintain elbow extension with the forearm held overhead
- Patients experiencing triceps muscle cramps on attempted activation

Preoperative assessment

Clinical assessment

Patient history

- The clinician should ascertain the mechanism of injury. This usually involves either a direct blow to the triceps tendon or an eccentric load applied to a contracting triceps
- A history of tobacco smoking and anabolic steroid use should be recorded
- A history of prodromal symptoms of posterior elbow pain suggestive of distal triceps tendinopathy should be documented

Physical examination

- Marked bruising and swelling of the posterior aspect of the elbow
- A palpable defect and tenderness just proximal to the olecranon process
- Proximal retraction of the triceps muscle belly
- Weakness of active elbow extension against gravity with the forearm held overhead
- A positive triceps squeeze test. The patient is asked to lie face down on the examining couch with the affected arm flexed to 90° over the edge of the couch. The clinician squeezes the triceps muscle belly. A triceps tendon rupture is indicated by an absence of passive elbow extension

Imaging assessment

Radiographs

- Plain anteroposterior and lateral radiographs may show flake avulsion fractures of the olecranon. Do not confuse calcific tendonitis with an avulsion fracture
- Radiographs are important to exclude olecranon fractures
- Olecranon spurs may suggest a pre-existing chronic tendinopathy

Ultrasound

- This is useful to diagnose a distal triceps tendon discontinuity
- It allows dynamic assessment of tendon patency
- Ultrasonography is, however, operator dependent, and interpretation of static scan images is difficult

Magnetic resonance imaging (MRI)

- Plain MRI is the most useful investigation. MRI will determine the pathoanatomy of a distal triceps tendon rupture accurately and will aid surgical planning
- Discontinuity of tendon structures can be seen. Wrinkling of the defunctioned tendon can be observed, as well as proximal retraction
- Sagittal and coronal T2-weighted images will be most useful in determining which of the three triceps heads is ruptured
- Typically, ruptures involve the long and lateral heads. The medial head lies deep to the others and is muscular almost to its insertion; it is therefore less prone to rupture

Timing for surgery

- Surgical repair should be performed as soon as possible, and certainly within 6 weeks of injury

- Beyond 3 weeks after the injury, there will be more formed scar tissue, and the retracted tendon will require greater dissection to mobilize it. The repair is more likely to require elbow extension to achieve tendon apposition to bone. This should not be a concern as the triceps stretches out over a few weeks of mobilization

Surgical preparation

Surgical equipment

- To achieve secure in-bone reduction and fixation of the avulsed triceps tendon, a round 5 mm high-speed burr and 2.5 mm drill are required
- A strong braided synthetic suture should be used. A no. 2 FiberLoop (Arthrex, Naples) is ideal for rapid whipstitch application, and the straight needle allows easy suture passage through bone tunnels
- If there are concerns regarding bone quality, a surgical button can be used to distribute the load of the suture repair over a greater cortical area

Equipment positioning

- A Mayo stand with a sterile cover is useful to rest the patient's extended arm on while performing the repair

Patient positioning

- Patient positioning depends on the surgeon's preference. The patient can be placed in a lateral decubitus position with the arm over a bolster. Alternatively, the patient can be positioned prone with the elbow flexed over the edge of the operating table, or supine with the arm across the chest
- Lateral positioning is facilitated by the use of a positioning suction beanbag (Snopak) and Trimano limb holder (Maquet) with elbow attachment (Arthrex)
- A high upper arm tourniquet should be applied

Further preparation

- Antibiotic prophylaxis according to local hospital policy should be administered prior to tourniquet inflation

Surgical technique

Exposure

- A posterior midline skin incision is made just lateral to the tip of the olecranon and continued up to the triceps
- Medial and lateral skin flaps are elevated. The position of the ulnar nerve is identified but it is not necessary to formally dissect the nerve out
- The torn end of the triceps tendon is identified and mobilized to allow a whipstitch to be placed
- The soft tissues are elevated from the medial and lateral sides of the ulna by sharp dissection for approximately 6 cm from the tip of the olecranon

Tendon repair

- A four-strand whipstitch is placed in the torn and retracted triceps tendon using two no. 2 FiberLoop (Arthrex) sutures (**Figure 4.1**)

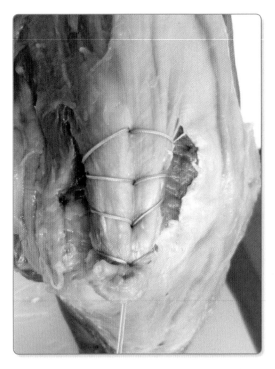

Figure 4.1 An Arthrex no. 2 FiberLoop suture in a torn long and lateral head triceps tendon avulsion.

- A trough is created at the footprint of the avulsed tendon on the olecranon using a 5 mm high-speed burr
- Using a 2.5 mm drill, two oblique bone tunnels are drilled in the olecranon from the medial point of the trough through the lateral cortex of the ulna, and from the lateral point of the trough through the medial cortex (**Figure 4.2**)
- A third transverse drill hole is created from the medial to the lateral cortex just distal to the exit point of the oblique tunnels (**Figure 4.3**)
- One end from each FiberLoop suture is passed through each oblique bone tunnel using the FiberLoop needle as a suture-passer (**Figure 4.4**)
- The suture ends that emerge on the medial side of the ulna are brought across the dorsum of the ulna and passed from lateral to medial through the transverse drill hole (**Figure 4.5**)
- These suture ends are then passed back across the dorsum of the ulna to the lateral side, where they are tied to the ends of the sutures emerging from the oblique lateral bone tunnel (**Figure 4.6**). The knot is then buried beneath the anconeus muscle to avoid soft tissue irritation (**Figure 4.7**)

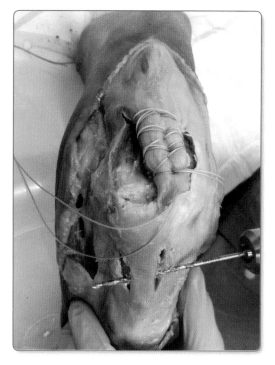

Figure 4.3 A third transverse drill hole is made with a 2.5 mm drill distal to the oblique bone tunnels.

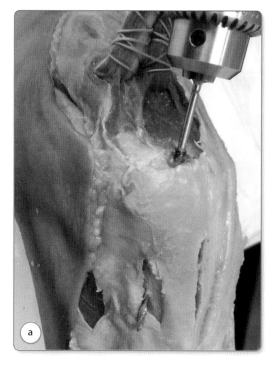

a

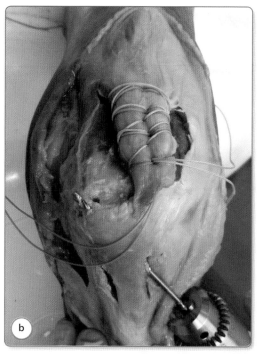

b

Figure 4.2 (a) and (b) Oblique bone tunnels are drilled with a 2.5 mm drill from the tip of the olecranon distally to exit the medial and lateral walls of the ulna about 6 cm from the tip.

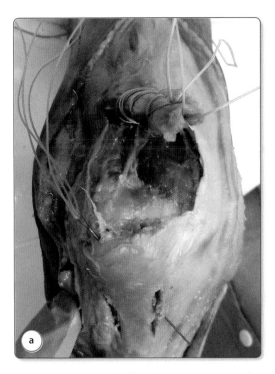
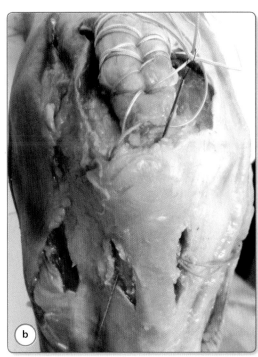

Figure 4.4 (a) The needle of the FiberLoop suture is used to pass the sutures through the bone tunnels. (b) One suture end from each pair of sutures is passed through each tunnel.

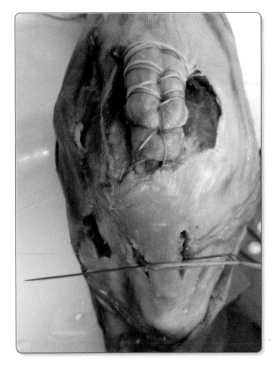
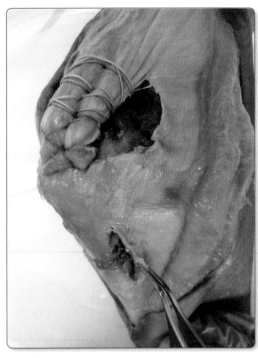

Figure 4.5 The sutures exiting from the medial bone tunnel are brought dorsally over the ulna and passed through the transverse bone tunnel.

Figure 4.6 The sutures are then passed back over the dorsum of the ulna and tied to the sutures on the lateral side.

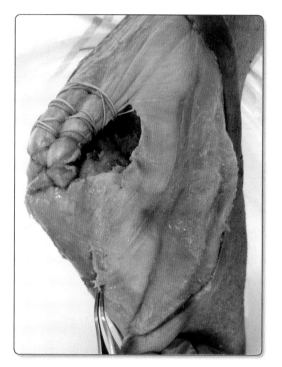

Figure 4.7 The suture knot is then buried beneath the anconeus to avoid irritation.

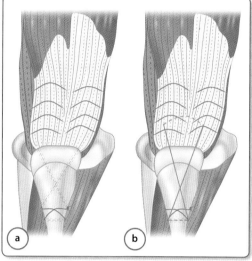

Figure 4.8 (a) Primary suture placement (blue). (b) Secondary footprint suture (green).

- An additional FiberWire suture is passed through the transverse bone tunnel and passed in the form of a cross through the triceps dorsally to provide additional fixation and to increase contact with the footprint (**Figure 4.8**)

Possible perioperative complications

- Iatrogenic ulnar nerve injury is possible
- Fracture of the ulna, resulting in fixation failure, is possible if the bone tunnels are placed too far dorsally
- As with other tendon repairs, re-rupture is possible and most commonly occurs early

Closure

- Layered closure is performed
- No drain is required, but the tourniquet should be deflated prior to closure and careful hemostasis achieved to avoid hematoma formation

Postoperative management

- A backslab should be applied across the extended elbow for 2 weeks postoperatively to allow the wound to heal without complications
- Isometric exercises should be undertaken with physiotherapy guidance while the elbow is still in plaster
- From 2 to 6 weeks, the patient can mobilize the elbow without loading
- From 6 to 12 weeks, gradual loading of the triceps is permitted building to full loading by the 12th postoperative week

Outpatient follow-up

- The patient should be reviewed at 2 weeks for wound inspection to ensure satisfactory wound healing
- A review at 6 weeks is required only if there is concern regarding the integrity of the repair

- Further imaging with ultrasonography or MRI is only required if there is reason to suspect re-rupture
- At the final 12-week review, the patient will be free to return to full activity as long as they have achieved 90% extension strength without pain. Ideally, isokinetic measurement is used to determine strength

Further reading

Paci JM, Clark J, Rizzi A. Distal triceps knotless anatomic footprint repair: a new technique. Arthrosc Tech 2014; 3:e621–e626.

Indications

- Reconstruction of a chronic distal triceps tendon rupture is indicated in patients with significant functional deficit due to weakness or pain
- A relative indication is the altered esthetics from proximal retraction of the muscle belly in body builders

Preoperative assessment

Clinical assessment

- Patients may also have other comorbidities such as renal failure requiring dialysis, diabetes, and smoking
- Inspection of the elbow may reveal scars from previous surgeries, e.g. bursectomy, olecranon osteosynthesis, or total elbow arthroplasty
- The triceps muscle belly is typically retracted proximally in a complete tear
- Delayed diagnosis of a triceps tendon rupture is likely to lead to muscle atrophy
- A gap may be visible or palpable between the olecranon and the triceps tendon stump, or the gap may be filled with fibrous tissue, making the diagnosis more difficult
- Both passive and active range of motion are noted
- Resisted extension of the elbow will demonstrate triceps weakness compared to the opposite side
- The ulnar nerve should be palpated and assessed for any pathology

Imaging assessment

Radiographs

- Anteroposterior and lateral views may show evidence of previous surgery such as retained metalwork or a total elbow replacement
- A bone flake proximal to the ulna indicates a bony triceps tendon avulsion, although this is not always present (**Figure 5.1**)

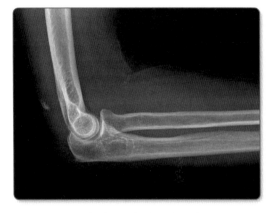

Figure 5.1   Lateral radiograph of an elbow showing a bone flake proximal to the ulna representing a bony triceps tendon avulsion. With permission from the MoRe Foundation.

- A traction spur indicates chronic triceps loading
- Calcification of the triceps tendon insertion may be noted, suggesting chronic tendinosis

Ultrasonography

- This modality is operator dependent, but may be helpful in the diagnosis of a triceps tendon rupture
- Other pathologies, e.g. tendinosis, inflammation, and calcification, can be identified
- It is sometimes difficult to differentiate between scar tissue and tendon, especially in post-surgical triceps tendon ruptures or delayed diagnoses

Magnetic resonance imaging (MRI)

- MRI will identify the position of the ruptured stump and the amount of proximal retraction (**Figure 5.2**)
- It is useful in cases where the clinical diagnosis is difficult due to the presence of fibrous scar tissue filling the gap
- The quality of the remaining tendon can be evaluated with MRI

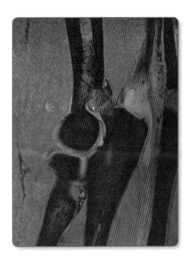

Figure 5.2 Saggital MRI showing a chronic triceps tendon rupture with retraction of the tendon stump. With permission from the MoRe Foundation.

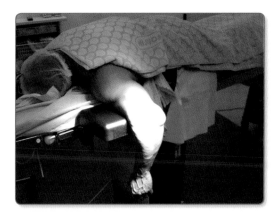

Figure 5.3 The patient is placed in the prone position, with the arm on a side support. Note that no tourniquet is used in chronic cases. With permission from the MoRe Foundation.

- The scan findings are useful for surgical planning; a partial tear or anconeus integrity may influence the operation choice, e.g. primary repair, anconeus turn-down flap, or allograft reconstruction

Timing for surgery

- Triceps tendon ruptures are best operated on as early as possible as this increases the chance of a successful primary repair
- Surgery within the first 3 weeks after injury gives superior results
- In delayed cases, the decision to proceed with reconstruction of the triceps is taken intraoperatively if primary repair is not possible

Surgical preparation

Surgical equipment

- Standard surgical instruments
- Power drill and 2.4 mm drill bit
- Suture retriever
- #2 nonabsorbable suture
- Bone anchors with non-resorbable sutures
- Achilles tendon allograft with a calcaneal bone block should be available for cases where primary repair will not be possible

Patient positioning

- Prone or lateral decubitus with the arm over a support (**Figure 5.3**)

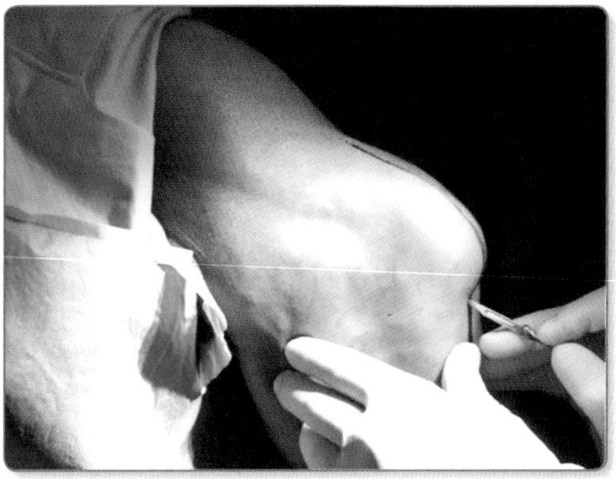

Figure 5.4 A midline posterior incision is used. With permission from the MoRe Foundation.

- A tourniquet is not used in chronic cases, as this would tether the triceps and limit the mobility of the retracted tendon
- The arm is prepped and draped all the way up to the shoulder

Surgical technique

- A longitudinal posterior midline incision is made (**Figure 5.4**)
- The ulnar nerve is identified and released to prevent nerve tethering when the tendon is later mobilized distally (**Figure 5.5**)
- All fibrous scar tissue is removed until healthy tendon becomes visible

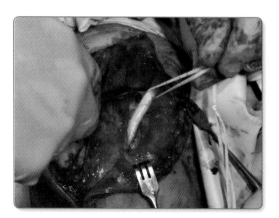

Figure 5.5 The ulnar nerve is usually surrounded by fibrous tissue from the chronic triceps tendon rupture. The nerve needs to be released and protected in order to prevent iatrogenic injury once the tendon stump is mobilized. With permission from the MoRe Foundation.

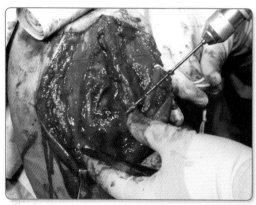

Figure 5.7 Oblique bone tunnels are drilled away from the ulnar nerve using a 2.5 mm drill bit. With permission from the MoRe Foundation.

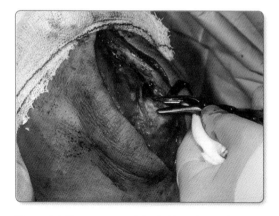

Figure 5.6 Fibrous tissue is debrided from the tendon stump. The olecranon tip is decorticated to promote ingrowth of the tendon. With permission from the MoRe Foundation.

- The olecranon tip is debrided to bleeding bone as this will facilitate tendon healing (**Figure 5.6**)
- The triceps tendon and muscle belly are released to mobilize the tendon sufficiently to reach the olecranon
- The elbow is extended to determine whether or not the tendon will reach the olecranon
- If the tendon reaches the olecranon, a primary repair may still be possible even in chronic cases. Otherwise, an allograft will have to be used to reconstruct the defect

Tendon fixation with primary repair to bone

- Using a 2.5 mm drill bit, two crossed diagonal bone tunnels are drilled in the proximal ulna (**Figure 5.7**). A third tunnel is drilled perpendicular to the ulna in order to achieve better fixation of the graft onto the proximal ulna
- The tunnels are drilled from medial to lateral to decrease the risk of iatrogenic ulnar nerve injury
- A suture retriever is used to pull two #2 nonabsorbable sutures through the tunnels (**Figure 5.8**)
- One or two bone anchors are drilled at the center of the olecranon tip for additional fixation
- The tendon is sutured with a running locked suture, using the #2 suture with the patient's arm in extension

Tendon reconstruction with an allograft

- The Achilles tendon allograft is prepared by first thawing it in physiologic fluid
- Any muscle residue is removed but it is important not to remove the calcaneal bone block at this stage
- The Achilles tendon allograft is wide and thin proximally, and narrow and thick toward the bone block; this ideally suits the natural anatomy of the triceps muscle aponeurosis defect

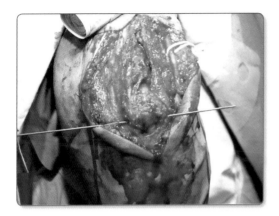

Figure 5.8 A suture retriever is used to pull a nonresorbable suture through the bone tunnel. With permission from the MoRe Foundation.

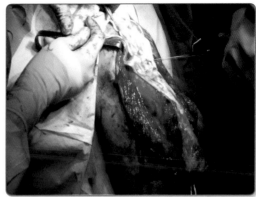

Figure 5.9 The Achilles tendon allograft is placed on the triceps tendon and securely sutured proximally and distally. The calcaneal bone is not removed until adequate proximal and distal fixation of the graft is confirmed. With permission from the MoRe Foundation.

Positioning and suturing of the allograft

- Extend the elbow and bring the triceps tendon stump as close to the olecranon as possible
- Place the Achilles tendon graft over the defect, with at least a further 5 cm overlapping the triceps proximally and the ulna distally
- If the olecranon bone quality is good, the allograft bone block will not be needed. In this case, place a thin but strong portion of the allograft over the subcutaneous border of the ulna
- In cases of olecranon bone loss or poor bone quality (e.g. rheumatoid arthritis, total elbow arthroplasty), the bone block can be used to fix the allograft bone block to the olecranon. The position of the bone block is determined at this stage
- Securely suture the proximal part of the allograft once the final position has been determined
- A three-row fixation is used. Suture the graft laterally, centrally, and medially to the triceps aponeurosis to avoid the accumulation of fluid between the graft and the triceps tendon

Fixation of the allograft with good bone quality

- Using a 2.5 mm drill bit, two crossed diagonal bone tunnels are drilled in the proximal ulna.

A third tunnel is drilled perpendicular to the ulna in order to achieve better fixation of the graft onto the proximal ulna
- The tunnels are drilled from medial to lateral to decrease the risk of iatrogenic ulnar nerve injury
- A suture retriever is used to feed the sutures through the bone tunnels
- With the elbow extended, the allograft–tendon unit is reduced to the olecranon and securely fixed (**Figure 5.9**)
- Suture knots should be buried in the muscle to avoid soft tissue irritation
- The bone block can now be removed, as can the thicker part of the graft distal to the fixation (**Figure 5.10**)

Fixation of the allograft with poor bone quality

- Proximal fixation of the allograft to the triceps is identical to the technique described above
- Bone tunnels are drilled as described above
- Using a high-speed burr, shape the calcaneal bone block so that it slides over the proximal ulna; the allograft bone block is placed 3–4 cm distally on the ulnar shaft, and not at the tip of the olecranon
- Two or three cerclage wires are used to secure the allograft bone block to the ulna (**Figure 5.11**)

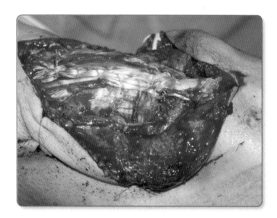

Figure 5.10 Good proximal and distal fixation of the Achilles tendon allograft. Note the low-profile reconstruction of the triceps tendon. With permission from the MoRe Foundation.

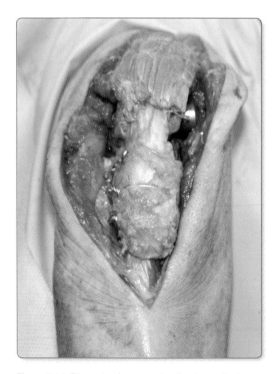

Figure 5.11 Triceps tendon reconstruction in a patient with rheumatoid arthritis following a total elbow replacement. The Achilles tendon graft is sutured to the remaining triceps, and the calcaneal bone is fixed to the proximal ulna with cerclage wires. With permission from the MoRe Foundation.

Testing the quality of the repair

- Move the elbow through a full range of flexion and extension to assess the integrity and the strength of the repair or reconstruction
- The repair or reconstruction can be reinforced at this stage, or alternatively postoperative flexion can be restricted to a tension-free range for a period of time
- The postoperative regimen is determined at this stage

Possible perioperative complications

- Ulnar nerve damage can be avoided by identifying, releasing, and protecting the nerve in all chronic cases
- Tunnel breakage can be avoided by creating tunnels that are long enough and have sufficient depth to withstand loading. Bone anchors can be used if tunnel breakage occurs. It is important not to drill the tunnels through the ulnar articulating surface
- In case of tendon slippage, increase the fixation strength with additional sutures or bone anchors
- If closing the skin over the bone block is difficult, decrease the volume of the bone block

Closure

- Close the subcutaneous layer with absorbable sutures followed by skin closure. Ensure all suture knots are buried to avoid soft tissue irritation or wound problems
- No drainage is required
- A simple dressing is applied
- The postoperative regimen is determined during the testing of the repair, and can include a protective bandage, immobilization, or dynamic bracing

Postoperative management

Postoperative regimen

- If the elbow can be moved freely without affecting the integrity of the repair or reconstruction through a full range of motion, only a protective bandage will be used. The patient will be allowed to flex the elbow actively at day 1 postoperatively as well as to try passive extension exercises. Passive flexion exercises must be avoided during the first 6 weeks

- When a tendon repair or reconstruction needs to be protected, the elbow can be immobilized in varying degrees of extension depending on the integrity and strength of the repair or reconstruction
- Most commonly, a dynamic elbow brace is used and flexion limited to 30° for 2 weeks, although full extension is permitted. Flexion is gradually increased, by 30° every 2 weeks, or slower if appropriate. Normally, full flexion is permitted after 6 weeks
- Ice packs are applied to reduce soft tissue swelling
- Analgesics medication is given regularly and as required, but non steroidal anti-inflammatory drugs are avoided due to the potential risk of impairment of tendon healing

Early-phase postoperative complications

- Swelling
- Deep or superficial wound infection

- Wound problems and breakdown due to possible suture knot irritation
- Ulnar nerve neuropathy
- Olecranon fracture

Late-phase postoperative complications

- Elbow stiffness, although almost 10° loss of the flexion–extension arc can be expected
- Ulnar neuropathy secondary to fibrosis around the nerve
- Re-rupture of the primary repair or allograft reconstruction
- Weakness of elbow extension

Outpatient follow-up

- Patients should be seen at 2 weeks to examine the wound and assess the neurovascular status
- A radiograph can be taken to check the bone tunnels and calcaneal bone block position
- Patients should be seen at 6 and 12 weeks to assess the elbow's range of motion
- Strength should be assessed after allograft integration at 12 weeks

Further reading

Celli A. Triceps tendon rupture: the knowledge acquired from the anatomy to the surgical repair. Musculoskeletal Surg 2015; 99:57–66.

Bennett JB, Mehlhoff TL. Triceps tendon repair. J Hand Surg 2015; 40:1677–1683.

van Riet RP, Morrey BF, Ho E, O'Driscoll SW. Surgical treatment of distal triceps ruptures. J Bone Joint Surg Am 2003; 85-A:1961–1967.

Indications

- Surgical repair of distal biceps tendon ruptures is indicated in all active patients who require strength and endurance of elbow flexion and supination

Preoperative assessment

Clinical assessment

There are two groups of patients that present with a distal biceps tendon rupture:

- The first group are typically men in their fourth or fifth decade with a complete tendon rupture following an acute trauma that usually involves a sudden extension force applied to a flexed elbow, resulting in an eccentric contraction of the biceps and a subsequent tearing sensation in the antecubital fossa. The normal biceps contour is lost and the 'popeye sign' may be present
- The second group are typically older patients with a chronic degenerative partial tendon rupture of insidious onset. These patients present with antecubital pain and weakness of elbow flexion and supination.The distal biceps tendon is still palpable on examination
- The hook test has a sensitivity and specificity of 100% to diagnose a distal biceps tendon rupture, and to distinguish between complete and partial ruptures:
  - When the distal biceps tendon is intact, the examiner can hook their index finger around the cord-like lateral edge of the tendon spanning the antecubital fossa in a flexed elbow
  - With a complete rupture, the hook test is positive, with the examiner unable to hook their finger around the tendon
  - With a partial rupture, the hook test is negative, with the examiner able to hook their finger around the tendon, but the test will result in pain

Imaging assessment

Radiographs

- Radiographs of the elbow can show some irregular bony changes or an avulsion at the radial bicipital tuberosity

Ultrasonography or magnetic resonance imaging (MRI)

- Ultrasonography and MRI may help diagnose distal biceps tendon ruptures but are mainly used to identify associated injuries and determine the retraction of the distal biceps tendon stump
- The flexed–abducted–supinated position of the elbow allows visualization of the entire length of the distal biceps tendon in only one or two MRI slices
- MRI is less accurate than the hook test in differentiating between a complete and a partial distal biceps tendon rupture

Timing for surgery

- Surgical reconstruction of the ruptured distal biceps tendon should be performed as soon as possible, preferably within 10 days of injury
- Several studies have reported more complications following late distal biceps tendon reconstructions compared to early surgery

Surgical preparation

Surgical equipment

- The necessary equipment for distal biceps tendon reconstructions depends on the type of reconstruction that will be performed. Generally there are four different options for reconstruction:
  - Suture anchors
  - Cortical buttons (**Figure 6.1**)
  - Interference screws (**Figure 6.2**)
  - Bone tunnels

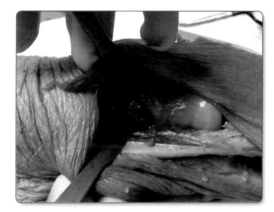

Figure 6.1 A demonstration of the endobutton technique in a cadaver.

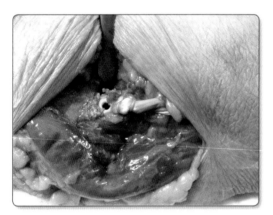

Figure 6.2 Interference screw technique in a cadaver.

- Different types of suture anchors, cortical buttons, and interference screws from various manufacturers have been described and may be used in accordance with the surgical techniques and accompanying instrumentation
- With bone tunnels, the use of strong nonabsorbable sutures is recommended
- A basic orthopaedic set, guidewires, and reamers of different diameters should be available

Equipment positioning

- Fluoroscopy is usually only used at the end of the surgical procedure, and the fluoroscopy equipment should be placed at the end of the hand table where it will not interfere with the positioning of the surgical team

Patient positioning

- The patient is placed in a supine position with the arm on a surgical hand table
- A sterile tourniquet is applied

Further preparation

- Implantation of material justifies antibiotic prophylaxis in accordance with local hospital policy and guidelines

Surgical technique

Exposure

Reconstruction of distal biceps tendon ruptures is performed by either a single incision anterior approach or a double-incision approach. It is important to appreciate the regional anatomy to ensure a safe and adequate exposure (**Figure 6.3**).

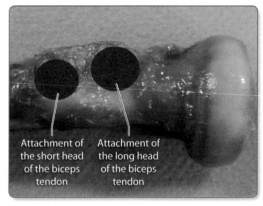

Attachment of the short head of the biceps tendon   Attachment of the long head of the biceps tendon

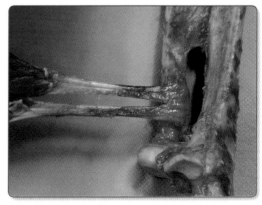

Figure 6.3 Distal biceps tendon double-footprint attachment at the radial bicipital tuberosity, and the surrounding anatomy in a cadaver.

- The single-incision anterior approach is as follows:
  - A 1 cm longitudinal incision is made from the elbow skin crease extending distally
  - The end of the distal biceps tendon is identified
  - A second more proximal incision over the end of the tendon may be needed to mobilize a retracted tendon stump
  - The lateral antebrachial cutaneous nerve (LABCN) is identified and protected throughout the procedure (**Figure 6.4**)
  - The LABCN runs with the cephalic vein on the anterolateral aspect of the elbow, and lies on the deep fascia within the deep adipose tissue
  - In chronic distal biceps tendon ruptures, the LABCN can become trapped in reactive inflammatory and scar tissue
  - Further blunt dissection at the proximal radius is performed with the brachioradialis retracted laterally, and the pronator teres retracted medially
  - The radial bicipital tuberosity is exposed with the elbow fully flexed and supinated

  - Debridement of the tendon footprint on the radial bicipital tuberosity and of the tendon stump are performed
  - In partial ruptures, the tear should be converted to a total rupture to allow adequate fixation of the whole tendon
- The double-incision approach is as follows:
  - A small transverse anterior antecubital incision is made
  - The end of the distal biceps tendon is identified
  - The radial bicipital tuberosity is palpated, and a curved clamp is passed just ulnar to the bicipital tuberosity into the interosseous space
  - The forearm is flexed, and a second incision is made over the posterolateral aspect of the elbow where the curved clamp is palpated
  - The proximal radius can be approached between the ulna and the anconeus, between the anconeus and the extensor carpi ulnaris, or between the extensor carpi ulnaris and the extensor digitorum communis
  - The posterior interosseous nerve (PIN) is not visualized as the laterally retracted supinator protects it (**Figure 6.5**)
  - The radial bicipital tuberosity is exposed by fully pronating the forearm

Tendon repair

- Suture anchors, cortical buttons, or interference screws are mainly used with a single incision anterior approach
- Bone tunnels or suture anchors are mainly used with a double-incision approach

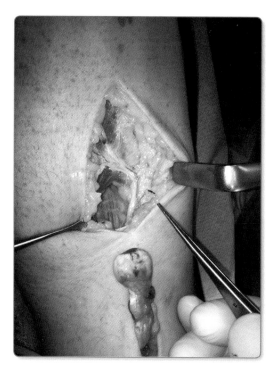

Figure 6.4 Identification of the lateral antebrachial cutaneous nerve.

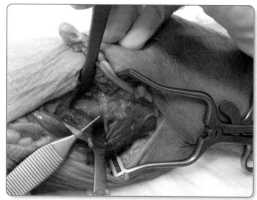

Figure 6.5 The anatomic relationship of the posterior interosseous nerve to the distal biceps tendon footprint.

- The following describes the cortical button reconstruction technique:
  - A guidewire is drilled into the anatomic footprint at the radial bicipital tuberosity. It is important to ensure the drill hole is in the correct rotational alignment
  - The guidewire should be aimed slightly distal and ulnar to angle away from the PIN
  - A 4.5 mm cannulated drill is advanced over the guidewire and through both cortices
  - The anterior cortex is subsequently drilled with a diameter based on the size of the debrided distal biceps tendon, which is usually 8 mm
  - A cortical button is fixed to the distal end of the biceps tendon
  - The cortical button is pulled through the radius using a Beath pin to pass the sutures
  - The cortical button is engaged on the posterior cortex and locked into place
  - The passing sutures are removed

Implant positioning

- Implant positioning should be as anatomic as possible, and should be confirmed using fluoroscopy

Possible perioperative complications

- Injury to the LABCN during the anterior approach can lead to a painful neuroma or paresthesia
- Injury to the PIN can occur during deep dissection of the proximal radius. Care should be taken when placing deep retractors and drilling the posterior cortex
- Most of the injuries to the PIN are neurapraxias that ultimately recover
- In chronic cases, the distal biceps tendon stump may have retracted and shortened to an extent requiring the use of an autograft or allograft interposition
- Re-rupture of the distal biceps tendon is rare, and is often the result of inadequate initial fixation or poor patient compliance

- Proximal placement of the reconstruction at the radial bicipital tuberosity can result in shortening of the moment arm or fracture through the radial neck. Fluoroscopy can be used to determine tunnel placement
- A tension slide technique overcomes possible inadequacy in suture length between the cortical button and the distal biceps tendon stump
- Heterotopic ossification is frequently seen following distal biceps tendon reconstructions and can sometimes lead to loss of motion
- Nonsteroidal anti-inflammatory drugs can be used as prophylaxis against heterotopic ossification although the evidence to support this is limited

Closure

- Close the subcutaneous and skin layers in a standard fashion
- No drainage is needed
- A long arm cast is applied with the elbow in flexion and the forearm in a neutral position

Postoperative management

- The elbow is immobilized in the cast for 1 week
- After the first week, physical therapy is commenced and both passive and active motion exercises are allowed
- Flexion against resistance is not allowed for the first 3 months
- After 3 months, patients are allowed to resume normal activities to pre-injury level

Outpatient follow-up

- Patients return for wound inspection and removal of sutures after 2 weeks
- Subsequent visits are after 6 weeks, 3 months, and 6 months
- Yearly follow-up visits can be arranged in order to evaluate the long-term outcome following distal biceps tendon reconstruction

Further reading

Cohen MS. Complications of distal biceps tendon repairs. Sports Med Arthrosc 2008; 16:148–153.

Miyamoto RG, Elser F, Millett PJ. Distal biceps tendon injuries. J Bone Joint Surg Am 2010; 92:2128–2138.

van den Bekerom MPJ, Kodde IF, Aster A, Bleys RL, Eygendaal D. Clinical relevance of distal biceps insertional and footprint anatomy. Knee Surg Sports Traumatol Arthrosc 2014 Sep 18. [Epub ahead of print].

Radial head fracture fixation

Indications

Indications for internal fixation of the radial head fractures are:

- Fractures displaced by more than 2 mm
- Fractures with a mechanical block to elbow joint movements

Preoperative assessment

Clinical assessment

- Patients describe localized elbow pain following a fall on the outstretched hand with the forearm in pronation
- On examination, assess for tenderness along the lateral aspect of the elbow. This may limit the range of motion of the elbow
- Examine the flexion and extension of the elbow, as well as the supination and pronation of the forearm, to determine the presence of a mechanical block. Aspiration of the joint hematoma is useful in evaluating the mechanical block, and it also reduces pain by decreasing the intra-articular pressure
- Examine the stability of the elbow by applying varus and valgus stress

Imaging assessment

Radiographs

- Anteroposterior and lateral views detect most radial head fractures. If no obvious fracture is identified, the presence of the fat pad sign may indicate a minimally displaced fracture. In addition, a radiocapitellar view and a modified lateral view of the elbow can be obtained with the tube angled at 45° toward the shoulder to detect subtle radial head fractures (**Figure 7.1**)

Computed tomography (CT)

- CT, especially with three-dimensional reconstruction, is very useful for comminuted fractures of the radial head to evaluate the fracture fragments and to plan the type of surgical fixation (**Figure 7.2**)

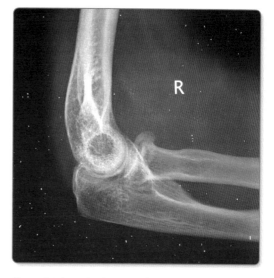

Figure 7.1 Lateral radiograph of the elbow showing a displaced radial head fracture.

Timing for surgery

- The operative procedure is performed once the edema around the elbow has settled

Surgical preparation

Surgical equipment

- A full selection of internal fixation and reconstructive options should be available as the most appropriate surgical procedure may change depending on the intraoperative findings
- The options for internal fixation include:
  - Various combinations of Kirschner wires for temporary fixation
  - Bioabsorbable screws, Herbert or Herbert-type screws, headless compression screws, and minifragment screws
  - Plates including T-plate, L-plate, and condylar blade plate
- The surgeon should be prepared to replace the radial head if indicated

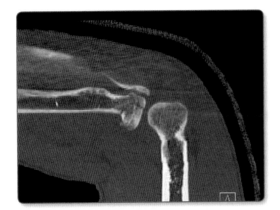

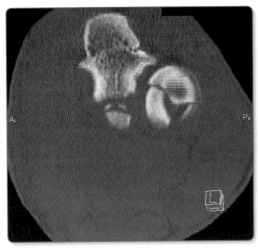

Figure 7.2 CT of the elbow showing greater detail of a radial head fracture, including the number of fracture fragments, the degree of fracture impaction, and their configuration.

- Complete hand set including lancet, forceps, Ragnell retractor, Baby Bennett retractor, curette, osteotomes, rongeur, pin cutter, reduction clamps, Kocher's forceps, and self-retaining retractors
- Diathermy apparatus
- Drill
- C-arm, which is essential for intraoperative fluoroscopy

Equipment positioning

- A tourniquet should be placed high in the arm and a fluoroscopy (a C-arm) should be available in the operating room

Patient positioning

- The patient is positioned supine with a sandbag under the ipsilateral scapula to facilitate the positioning of the hand across the chest. Alternatively, a hand table is used to support the upper extremity
- A pneumatic tourniquet is applied to the upper arm. A sterile tourniquet provides a better operative view. The limb is exsanguinated with an Esmarch bandage or simple arm elevation and the tourniquet inflated to 250 mmHg, approximately 100–120 mmHg above the systolic blood pressure

Further preparation

- Implantation of materials justifies antibiotic prophylaxis according to local hospital policy and guidelines, approximately 30 minutes before the incision. The author uses a second-generation cephalosporin, with an additional antibiotic dose administered postoperatively

Anesthesia

- General anesthesia enables immediate postoperative neurologic assessment
- Nerve blocks, e.g. interscalene nerve block, axillary brachial plexus block, or peripheral nerve block, allows better postoperative analgesia

Surgical technique

Exposure

- For isolated radial head fractures, a posterolateral approach to the elbow (Kocher's approach) is preferred
- An alternative lateral approach to the elbow (Kaplan's approach) is also described below

Posterolateral approach to the elbow (Kocher's approach)

- Begin the skin incision proximally from the lateral epicondyle and extend it distally over the radial head, which is palpable with pronation and supination of the forearm. The skin incision can be longitudinal or mildly curved and is approximately 5 cm (**Figure 7.3**)
- Incise the fascia between the anconeus and the extensor carpi ulnaris (ECU). Keeping the dissection parallel to the ECU fibers

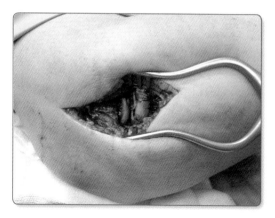

Figure 7.3 Posterolateral approach to the elbow (Kocher's approach).

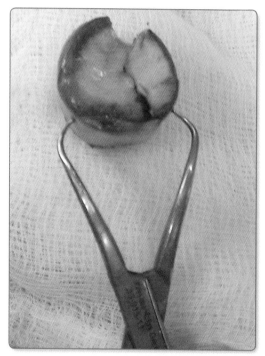

Figure 7.4 Anatomic reduction of the fragments is facilitated with gentle application of reduction clamps.

preserves the ECU fascial contributions to the posterolateral ligamentous complex. The ECU is retracted anteriorly, and an incision is then made in the joint capsule anterior to the lateral ligamentous structures. Avoid dissecting the joint capsule distally or anteriorly to avoid injuring the posterior interosseous nerve (PIN), which passes beneath the radial neck

- Keeping the arm pronated during this dissection avoids injury to the PIN
- Incise the annular ligament with a 'Z' cut and expose the fracture fragments
- The most appropriate surgical procedure is decided at this stage
- If the lateral ligamentous complex demonstrates injury or avulsion, a running locking suture is placed in the fibers, to protect them for later repair

Lateral approach to the elbow (Kaplan's approach)

- Begin the skin incision proximal to the lateral epicondyle and extend it distally across the radiocapitellar joint
- The plane between the extensor carpi radialis brevis and the extensor digitorum communis is developed
- Expose the supinator muscle and detach the ulnar and humeral heads of the supinator to expose the annular ligament
- Incise the annular ligament to expose the fracture fragments of the radial head
- Keep the arm pronated during this approach in order to avoid injury to the PIN, which runs approximately 2 cm below the radial head

Fracture reduction

- Identify the radial head fracture fragments, carefully maintaining any soft tissue attachments. Reduction clamps are gently applied to achieve provisional fixation of the articular surface of the radial head
- Kirschner wires can be used for temporary fixation of the fragments
- In cases where reduction cannot be achieved, the surgeon can remove the fragments from the joint and attempt provisional fixation of the radial head on the hand table (**Figures 7.4** and **7.5**). The radial head can then be fixed to the radial neck with a plate and additional screws

Implant positioning

- Place the metalwork posterolaterally in the safe zone to prevent impingement on the proximal radioulnar joint. The safe zone is within a 90–110° arc between the radial styloid and the dorsal tubercle of the radius, with the forearm in neutral rotation
- For fractures that do not involve the radial neck, fixation can be achieved with small screws such as Acutrak screws, Herbert screws,

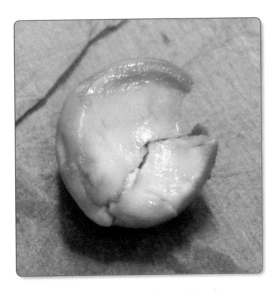

Figure 7.5 Provisional fixation of the radial head is performed with mini-fragment screws before the final fixation of the radial head to the radial neck.

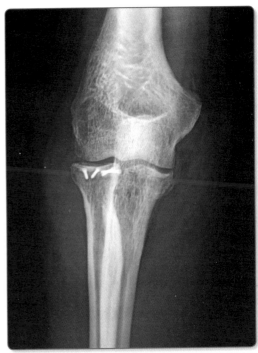

Figure 7.7 Internal fixation of a radial head fracture with four mini-fragment screws.

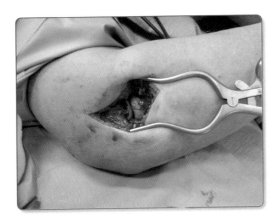

Figure 7.6 Fixation of a radial head fracture with mini-fragment screws. The screws are placed beneath the articular surface.

mini-fragment screws (1.5, 2.0, or 2.7 mm), or cannulated screws (3.0 mm) (**Figure 7.6**)
- The screws are placed beneath the articular surface to support it from collapse. The screws should not penetrate the opposite cortex, and should be countersunk to avoid any prominence. The Herbert screws can be placed in the articular surface of the radial head, deep in the cartilage. Multiple screws can be inserted obliquely through the head fragment into the neck to obtain compression and a stable reduction. A minimum of two screws in orthogonal planes is recommended to maintain rotational control in fractures with large fragments (**Figures 7.7** and **7.8**)
- For fractures that involve the radial neck, it is often essential to use mini T-plates for definitive fixation; these sometimes require bone grafting to elevate the articular surface of the radial head (**Figures 7.9** and **7.10**)
- The use of Kirschner wires as definitive fixation is not recommended because they tend to migrate postoperatively and impinge on adjacent soft tissues and bone

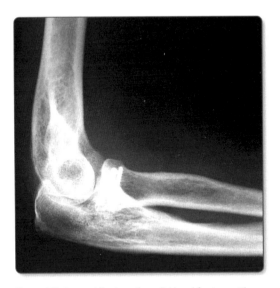

Figure 7.8 Internal fixation of a radial head fracture with two 3 mm screws.

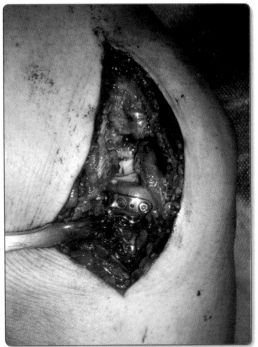

Figure 7.9 Reconstruction of a comminuted radial head and neck fracture with a mini-plate and screws.

Possible perioperative complications

- Injury to the PIN is more likely with the lateral (Kaplan's) approach to the elbow
- Injury to the lateral ligamentous complex is more likely with the posterolateral (Kocher's) approach to the elbow
- Failure of fixation
- Loss of forearm rotation due to proximal radioulnar impingement

Closure

- The wound must be irrigated and then closed in layers
- It is important to close the annular ligament and repair the lateral ligamentous complex to prevent instability
- Close the subcutaneous and skin layers in a standard fashion
- A simple dressing is applied
- Use a drain for 24 hours and immobilize the arm in a posterior splint

Postoperative management

- Analgesics are given orally or intramuscularly. Nonsteroidal anti-inflammatory drugs should be administered with caution as they may interfere with fracture healing
- The surgeon has to individualize the postoperative rehabilitation based on the fracture configuration and internal fixation stability
- If the fracture is deemed stable at the end of the surgical procedure, mobilization can commence in the first 24–48 hours
- In all cases, the splint should not be used for more than 7 days. The mobilization of the elbow includes:
  - Active movement, where the elbow is moved by the patient through the contraction of the arm muscles
  - Active assisted movement, where the elbow is moved through the contraction of the arm muscles and assistance is applied externally by the therapist or by the patient using their other hand

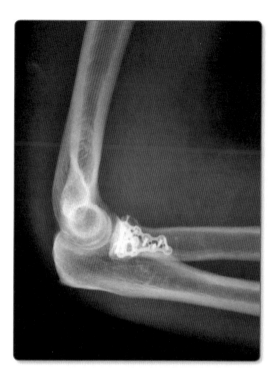

Figure 7.10 A lateral radiograph of the elbow showing anatomic reduction and stable fixation of a comminuted radial head fracture with a miniplate and screws.

– Passive movement, where the elbow is moved by the therapist or by the patient using their other hand

Outpatient follow-up

- Outpatient follow-up is at days 30, 60, and 90 with radiographs to check fracture union

Postoperative complications

- Infection
- Failure of fixation
- Limitation of forearm rotation
- Stiffness of the elbow with decreased flexion and/or extension
- Radiocapitellar joint arthritis
- Heterotopic ossification

Implant removal

- Metalwork removal is not required unless there is a complication such as infection or impingement of the proximal radioulnar joint due to the metalwork

Further reading

Ditsios KT, Stavridis SI, Christodoulou AG. The effect of haematoma aspiration on intra-articular pressure and pain relief following Mason I radial head fractures. Injury 2011; 42:362–365.

Jackson JD, Steinmann SP. Radial head fractures. Hand Clin 2007; 23:185–193.

Smith AM, Morrey BF, Steinmann SP. Low profile fixation of radial head and neck fractures: surgical technique and clinical experience. J Orthop Trauma 2007; 21:718–724.

Ring D, Quintero J, Jupiter JP. Open reduction and internal fixation of fractures of the radial head. J Bone Joint Surg Am 2002; 84-A:1811–8115.

Prosthetic radial head replacement

Indications

- Prosthetic radial head replacement is indicated in patients with an acute nonreconstructible radial head fracture in conjunction with elbow dislocation or instability
- Chronic indications are rare but may include a nonunion or malunion of a radial head or neck fracture, a missed Essex-Lopresti injury, or valgus instability following radial head resection

Preoperative assessment

Clinical assessment

- Inspection of the elbow will identify swelling and bulging at the soft spot
- A hematoma may be present on the lateral or medial side of the elbow, indicating a collateral ligament injury
- The forearm can be painful to palpation in the presence of an interosseous membrane injury
- Both passive and active range of motion of the elbow are recorded:
  - Flexion and extension are reduced secondary to hemarthrosis
  - Pronation and supination are reduced secondary to pain, but a mechanical block to rotation may be present
- The wrist is examined for fractures or triangular fibrocartilagenous complex injury at the distal radioulnar joint
- Pain limits stability testing in acute cases, but is an important part of the clinical examination in chronic cases

Imaging assessment

Radiographs

- Anteroposterior and lateral views of the elbow will show a comminuted radial head fracture
- Displacement of the fragments is correlated to the severity of the injury
- Carefully assess the presence of any associated bony lesions

- Subtle or gross signs of instability may be present
- Check for signs of previous injury or osteoarthritis
- A posterior fat pad sign confirms the presence of hemarthrosis
- Anteroposterior and lateral views of the wrist may show an associated scaphoid fracture or distal radioulnar joint dissociation with proximal radial migration

Computed tomography (CT)

- Minimally displaced fractures on plain radiographs may show significant displacement on CT
- CT is the most useful imaging modality to identify the number of fracture fragments, and their configuration and displacement
- Associated lesions not visible or difficult to assess on plain radiographs are readily visible with CT
- Three-dimensional reconstructions of CT data can help preoperative planning and counseling of the patient (**Figure 8.1**)

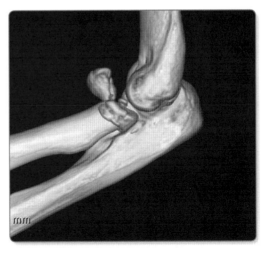

Figure 8.1 CT 3D reconstruction of an unreconstructable radial head fracture. With permission from the MoRe Foundation.

Magnetic resonance imaging (MRI)

- MRI will identify associated soft tissue lesions, although this does not influence the treatment in acute cases
- MRI is not recommended in the acute setting but may be helpful in chronic cases

Timing for surgery

- Comminuted radial head fractures are preferably operated on as soon as possible

Surgical preparation

Surgical equipment

- Standard surgical instruments
- Oscillating power saw
- Irrigation fluid and suction
- A prosthesis of choice that the surgeon is familiar with. There are a number of options, including:
  - Modular fixed monopolar design
  - Modular loose-fit monopolar design
  - Bipolar radial head design
  - Cemented or uncemented prostheses
- The following equipment may sometimes also be needed:
  - Bone anchors
  - Bone cement for cemented prostheses
  - Additional screws or plates to treat associated lesions
  - Fluoroscopy

Patient positioning

- Supine position with the arm on an arm table
- Positioning to ensure ease of access of fluoroscopy
- General anesthesia with additional local regional anesthesia with an ultrasound-guided supraclavicular block, depending on patient preference
- Antibiotic prophylaxis in accordance with local hospital policy and guidelines, administered prior to tourniquet inflation
- Exsanguination and application of a tourniquet at 250 mmHg
- It may be useful to elevate the elbow with a pack of swabs on the arm table
- Preparation and draping of the arm up to the tourniquet

Surgical technique

- With the arm fully pronated to protect the posterior interosseous nerve (PIN), a 4–5 cm incision is made on the lateral side of the elbow
- The incision is slightly curved and centered over the radial head and lateral epicondyle of the humerus. Distally, the incision heads towards Lister's tubercle
- Palpate the lateral collateral ligament (LCL). The LCL, and sometimes the extensor tendon mass, may be avulsed from the lateral epicondyle in comminuted radial head fractures
- An extensor tendon split from possible soft tissue tearing is used to gain access to the joint. Otherwise split the extensor tendon mass longitudinally in line with and directly anterior to the LCL (**Figure 8.2**)
- Release the lateral part of the anterior capsule from the anterior humeral cortex
- Divide the annular ligament sharply and in line with the extensor tendon split, and tag with a suture to aid closure
- Evacuate and rinse the fracture hematoma
- Evaluate the fracture fragments:
  - The final decision to replace the radial head with a prosthesis is taken at this point
  - A radial head prosthesis is used if the radial head fracture is considered to be nonreconstructible
- Remove all fragments and repeat the irrigation (**Figure 8.3**)

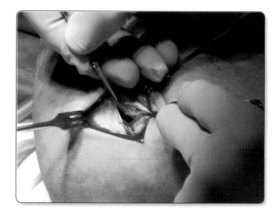

Figure 8.2 Split the extensor tendon mass anterior to the lateral collateral ligament. With permission from the MoRe Foundation.

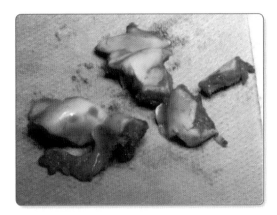

Figure 8.3 Excised radial head fragments. With permission from the MoRe Foundation.

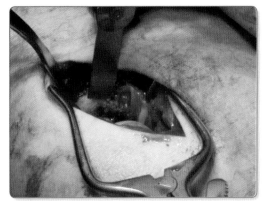

Figure 8.4 Radial neck osteotomy with an oscillating saw. With permission from the MoRe Foundation.

- Perform a neck osteotomy with a sagittal saw just proximal to the fracture. It is important not to resect too much bone (**Figure 8.4**)
- Most prostheses will reconstruct up to 20 mm of radial neck and head
- If access to the intramedullary canal is difficult, a varus stress and supination can improve visibility
- Ream the intramedullary canal to the appropriate size with the forearm held in neutral, ensuring that the radial tuberosity is medial (**Figure 8.5**)
- Ensuring that the radial tuberosity is medial improves the view of the intramedullary canal as this allows the neck to point laterally
- If a retractor is used to elevate the radial neck, care must be taken to avoid iatrogenic injury to the PIN
- The neck osteotomy cut should be perpendicular to the neck, but this can be fine-tuned with a collared reamer

Size and position of the prosthesis

- The radial head size should be estimated from the excised fracture fragments that can be reconstructed on the arm table
- If the radial head size falls between two sizes, select the smaller size
- Use of a modular system will optimize the correct bony fit and soft tissue tension
- Rasp the bone until the prosthesis is a tight fit in the radial neck
- The height of the collar should now be estimated to ensure restoration of the anatomic radial length (**Figure 8.6**)

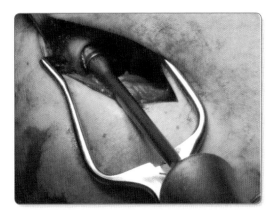

Figure 8.5 Reaming of the radial neck intramedullary canal. With permission from the MoRe Foundation.

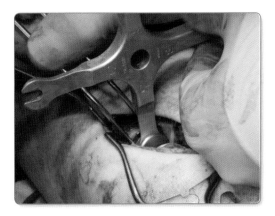

Figure 8.6 The height of the radial head replacement assessed using a tool offering different heights. With permission from the MoRe Foundation.

- It is important to get the length of the prosthesis right, especially in the presence of an LCL avulsion, where it is easy to overstuff the joint
- The head of the prosthesis should sit flush in the sigmoid notch of the ulna, which it would articulate with

Trialing the prosthesis

- Trial a suitably sized radial head and length of collar that restores radial length
- Move the elbow through a full range of flexion, extension, supination, and pronation, and assess elbow stability
- The prosthesis should articulate comfortably with the capitellum throughout the range of motion, but some translation will occur with supination and pronation
- To avoid overstuffing the joint, the most proximal part of the radial head should sit at the level of the coronoid on a lateral fluoroscopy view (**Figure 8.7**)

Testing stability of the elbow

- Assess elbow stability with varus and valgus stressing under continuous screening fluoroscopy
- If the prosthesis is too long, the joint will tilt into varus

- If the prosthesis is too short, the joint will tilt into valgus

Definitive placement of the prosthesis

- With an uncemented prosthesis, a secure press-fit is required. It is important to be careful not to fracture the radial neck on impaction
- The arm should be held in a neutral position when inserting the prosthesis
- Usually the laser marking on the prosthesis points laterally and signifies the long axis of the elliptical shape of the radial head. This mark should point towards Lister's tubercle (**Figure 8.8**)
- The prosthesis stem needs to be tapped into the medullary canal of the radial neck firmly to obtain a good press-fit (**Figure 8.9**)
- If the LCL has been avulsed, one or two bone anchors are inserted at the isometric point of the lateral epicondyle, and nonabsorbable running locked sutures are used to repair the ligament
- If the radial head fracture is part of a 'terrible triad' coronoid fractures and the medial collateral ligament complex may also require repair once the radial length has been recreated and the LCL repaired

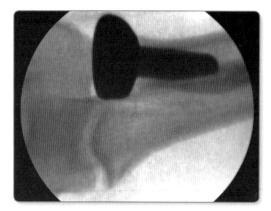

Figure 8.7 Fluoroscopy can be used to evaluate the position of the radial head prosthesis. With permission from the MoRe Foundation.

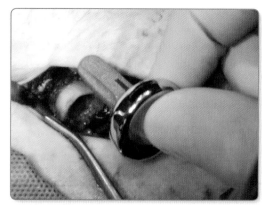

Figure 8.8 A laser mark on the radial head prosthesis to allow correct orientation. As this particular design has an elliptical, anatomic shape, it is important to ensure the orientation is correct. With permission from the MoRe Foundation.

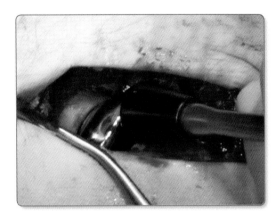

Figure 8.9 The stem of the radial head prosthesis is inserted tightly in the radial neck. With permission from the MoRe Foundation.

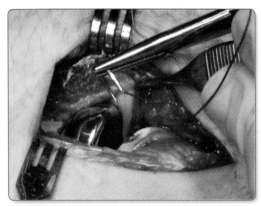

Figure 8.10 Closure of the annular ligament. With permission from the MoRe Foundation.

Possible perioperative complications

- Fracture of the radial neck could be associated with the original injury or sustained on impacting the prosthesis. A cerclage wire can be used to stabilize the fracture if a radial neck split occurs
- Pullout of anchors can be managed by replacing the anchors or using bone tunnels with transosseous sutures to fix the LCL complex
- Over- or understuffing of the joint should be avoided, as should over- and underlengthening of the radius. Changing the size or position of the prosthesis usually deals with this complication
- PIN injury may occur with forearm supination or the use of retractors around the radial neck

Closure

- The annular ligament is closed over the prosthesis with an absorbable suture (**Figure 8.10**)
- The extensor tendon split is closed (**Figure 8.11**), and the LCL repaired as necessary
- Standard subcutaneous and skin closure is performed
- No drainage is required
- A compressive bandage is applied for 2 weeks, but if an LCL repair has been performed, a removable 90° elbow splint is used

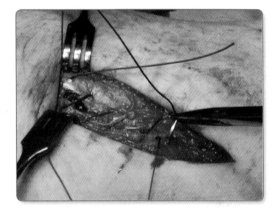

Figure 8.11 The extensor tendon split is closed using absorbable suture. With permission from the MoRe Foundation.

Postoperative management

Postoperative regimen

- Analgesic medication is required
- Physiotherapy referral is made; the protocol depends on the integrity of the LCL:
  - Intact LCL: compressive bandage, active and passive extension and flexion permitted immediately
  - LCL repair: splint removed and changed to a dynamic elbow brace the day after surgery
    - Flexion is free and extension is blocked to 60° of flexion

- Active and passive extension and flexion are permitted immediately within the range of the brace
- Extension is increased by 30° every 2 weeks
- The brace is discontinued after 6 weeks

Early-phase complications

- Swelling
- Wound dehiscence
- Deep infection
- Decreased strength
- Residual instability

Late-phase complications

- Loosening of the prosthesis
- Radial neck osteolysis
- Erosion of the capitellum
- Osteoarthritic changes in the elbow
- Heterotopic ossification
- Stiffness

Outpatient follow-up

- The patient is seen at 2 weeks for suture removal and radiography (**Figure 8.12**)

- Radiographic follow-up is at 3 months and yearly thereafter to check for implant loosening

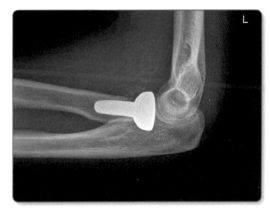

Figure 8.12 Postoperative lateral radiograph of the elbow showing a well-positioned radial head prosthesis and a congruent joint. With permission from the MoRe Foundation.

Further reading

Acevedo DC, Paxton ES, Kukelyansky I, Abboud J, Ramsey M. Radial head arthroplasty: state of the art. J Am Acad Orthop Surg 2014; 22:633–642.

Bain GI, Ashwood N, Baird R, Unni R. Management of Mason type-III radial head fractures with a titanium prosthesis, ligament repair, and early mobilization. Surgical technique. J Bone Joint Surg Am 2005; 87:136–147.

van Riet RP, van Glabbeek F. History of radial head prosthesis in traumatology. Acta Orthop Belg 2007; 73:12–20.

van Riet RP, van Glabbeek F, de Weerdt W, Oemar J, Bortier H. Validation of the lesser sigmoid notch of the ulna as a reference point for accurate placement of a prosthesis for the head of the radius: a cadaver study. J Bone Joint Surg Br 2007; 89:413–416.

Indications

- Olecranon fracture open reduction internal fixation (ORIF) is indicated in active patients, irrespective of fragment displacement, to allow early mobilization and rehabilitation. This includes Monteggia variants, elbow instability, and frank dislocation
- Depending on the patients' comorbidities, conservative treatment may be appropriate in elderly patients with non- or minimally displaced fractures. ORIF is, however, also indicated in elderly patients with displaced olecranon fractures
- Other indications for ORIF include painful nonunion or malunion, or following elective osteotomy

Preoperative assessment

Clinical assessment

- An obvious deformity of the elbow will often be present in displaced olecranon or proximal ulnar fractures, as well as in fracture–dislocations
- Inspection of the elbow will identify any swelling and hematoma
- Hemorrhagic bursitis may be present
- Bulging at the soft spot of the elbow indicates an intra-articular hematoma
- Medial or lateral hematomas may indicate concomitant collateral ligament damage or radial head or neck fracture
- The skin should be inspected for abrasions, wounds, and blisters that may require surgery to be postponed until the soft tissues settle
- The presence of bleeding around the elbow should raise the probability of an open fracture, and antibiotic prophylaxis according to local hospital policy and guidelines should be administered
- The subcutaneous border of the olecranon should be palpated; a depression may indicate a displaced fracture

- Distal neurovascular status should be recorded, paying particular attention to the ulnar nerve's sensory and motor branches
- If possible, both passive and active ranges of movement are noted. Weakness of extension may indicate a disruption of the extensor apparatus
- The wrist and shoulder should also be examined to rule out any concomitant ipsilateral injuries

Imaging assessment

Radiographs

- Standard anteroposterior and lateral radiographs usually identify the fracture
- Displacement of the fracture may indicate disruption of the extensor apparatus
- Radiographs should be scrutinized for intra-articular comminution and fragments, and fracture configuration

Computed tomography (CT)

- CT is indicated if intra-articular extension is suspected or the fracture configuration is not clearly defined
- Scans should be assessed for the presence of arthritis and any previous injuries
- CT may be useful to exclude complex fractures of the elbow, and will readily demonstrate comminution and fracture line obliquity
- CT may also help with preoperative counseling of the patient

Magnetic resonance imaging (MRI)

- MRI has no role for these bony injuries

Timing for surgery

- Surgery should be carried out as soon as the soft tissues settle to allow early mobilization and prevent postoperative stiffness
- In patients with an open fracture of the olecranon, an acute washout and debridement may be performed first, with a delayed second-stage definitive ORIF procedure

Surgical preparation

Surgical equipment

- Standard surgical equipment
- Fracture reduction forceps
- Motorized drill and 2.5 mm drill bit
- Fluoroscopy, positioned at the head of the patient
- Tension band plate and screws of different sizes
- 1.5 mm Kirschner wires

Patient positioning

- Either the lateral decubitus or prone position is appropriate
- The operative arm is allowed to hang free over padded support
- Ensure ease of access for fluoroscopy before preparation and draping the arm
- General anesthesia is administered with additional local regional anesthesia using an ultrasound-guided supraclavicular block, depending on the patient's preference
- Antibiotic prophylaxis is administered according to local hospital policy and guidelines prior to tourniquet inflation
- A more proximal position of the tourniquet that will not interfere with fracture reduction is preferred. The arm is exsanguinated and the tourniquet inflated to 250 mmHg
- The arm is prepared and draped up to the tourniquet
- The forearm can be draped separately as an added antiseptic measure or, if excessive swelling is expected, to decrease the chances of compartment syndrome

Surgical technique

- The authors' preferred method of fixation is a precontoured limited-contact dynamic compression plate, but tension band wiring can often be used in these fractures. Significantly comminuted or more distal fractures of the proximal ulna that are not amenable to tension band plating should be managed with longer bridging plates, with three screws distal to the fracture for stable cortical fixation

Exposure

- A 6 cm longitudinal posterior midline incision is made over the subcutaneous border of the olecranon, centered over the fracture (**Figure 9.1**)
- The incision may be curved radially over the olecranon tip to reduce the risk of a sensitive scar or wound breakdown
- Minimal sharp dissection is performed through the bursa and triceps paratenon
- Thick medial and lateral soft tissue flaps are minimally elevated
- If a more bulky plate is used, the extensor and flexor carpi ulnaris can be minimally undermined submuscularly to allow better plate seating on the proximal ulna. This is not usually necessary with the plate described below
- Proximally, the incision should extend far enough to allow fracture fragment manipulation without significant soft tissue tension

Fracture reduction

- The fracture is debrided and the intra-articular hematoma irrigated. Any interposing soft tissue is excised (**Figure 9.2**)
- Assess fracture comminution and any intra-articular extension carefully
- The fracture may be reduced directly with digital manipulation or using fracture reduction forceps
- Extending the elbow will make it easier to reduce the fracture fragments as this decreases tension in the extensor apparatus
- In comminuted cases, the fracture fragments may be temporarily held with parallel 1.5 mm Kirschner wires

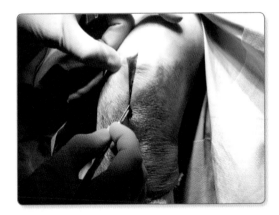

Figure 9.1 Posterior midline incision over the proximal ulna. With permission of the MoRe Foundation.

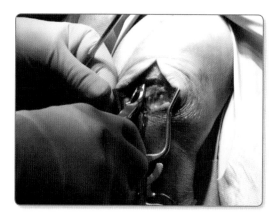

Figure 9.2 Fracture debridement with bone nibblers. With permission of the MoRe Foundation.

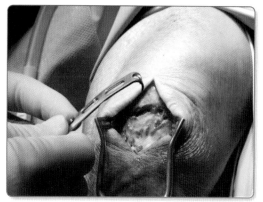

Figure 9.3 A precontoured, limited-contact dynamic compression tension band plate. With permission of the MoRe Foundation.

- If Kirschner wires are used, it is important to ensure they do not hinder the position of the plate

Plate application

- The authors' preferred method of fixation is a pre-contoured limited-contact dynamic compression tension band plate (**Figure 9.3**)
- The tension band plate is applied to the distal ulna with its hooks over the triceps tendon at the proximal olecranon
- The olecranon can be predrilled in hard bone to accommodate the hooks of the plate, but in soft bone the hooks can be simply pushed in
- Using a 2.5 mm drill bit, drill the oval sliding hole of the plate distally to allow compression at the fracture site (**Figure 9.4**)
- Measure the screw length and insert a nonlocking 3.5 mm screw, into the hole
- Do not fully tighten the screw but make sure the screw has sufficient purchase to compress the fracture later
- A longer temporary bicortical screw can be used in osteoporotic bone for added stability. Although the screw will lie proud of the anterior cortex of the proximal ulna, it can be changed to a shorter screw at the end of the procedure
- Using pointed fracture reduction forceps between the screw and the proximal olecranon, further compress the fracture site if comminution allows (**Figure 9.5**)
- With the fracture compressed, drill a second hole using the 2.5 mm drill bit in the distal hole of the plate

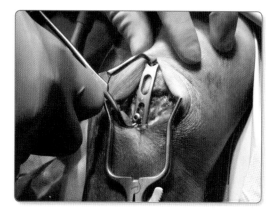

Figure 9.4 The first screw is placed in the sliding hole. With permission of the MoRe Foundation.

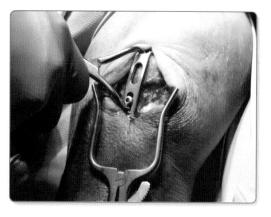

Figure 9.5 Fracture reduction using a reduction clamp. Note the change in position of the plate relative to the screw. With permission of the MoRe Foundation.

- Measure and insert a 3.5 mm screw in the second hole just drilled (**Figure 9.6**). Tighten both screws to hold the fracture in a compressed position
- Fracture reduction and stability are tested using fluoroscopy
- If fluoroscopy is satisfactory, a bicortical 'home-run' screw is inserted through the proximal hole in the plate after drilling (**Figures 9.7** and **9.8**)
- Drilling of the home-run screw can be done under direct fluoroscopic view, ensuring it is placed in the subchondral bone and not intra-articularly (**Figure 9.9**)
- Under fluoroscopic control, the elbow is put through a full range of movement, and elbow stability is tested with varus and valgus stress
- If a longer temporary screw was used for compression in osteoporotic bone, this can now be changed for a screw of the appropriate size

Possible perioperative complications

- Care should be taken not to narrow the trochlear groove in cases of sigmoid notch comminution as this will lead to joint incongruency and secondary osteoarthritis
- The plate should be placed directly over the olecranon to avoid ulnohumeral and proximal radioulnar intra-articular screw penetration

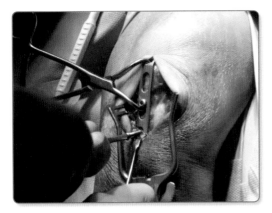

Figure 9.6 A second screw is inserted distally. With permission of the MoRe Foundation.

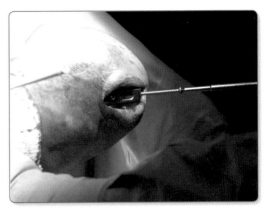

Figure 9.8 The home-run screw inserted. With permission of the MoRe Foundation.

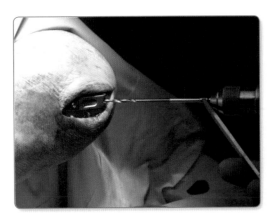

Figure 9.7 The home-run screw drilled. With permission of the MoRe Foundation.

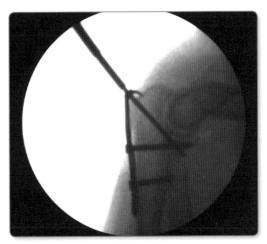

Figure 9.9 The position of the home-run screw is checked using fluoroscopy. With permission of the MoRe Foundation.

- The chances of proximal radioulnar joint screw penetration may be reduced with precontoured plates and drill guides. If a noncontoured plate is used, angling the screws medially avoids intra-articular screw penetration
- Ulnar neuropathy can be caused by metalwork or iatrogenic injury
- Median artery and nerve injury can result from anterior cortical screw penetration
- Ulnohumeral instability can be seen after plate fixation
- Insufficient proximal fixation can be caused by comminution of the proximal fragments. An unloading triceps suture placed under the hooks of the plate and into the triceps tendon approximately 3 cm from the plate will decrease tension on the ORIF construct. Tightening the suture loop decreases tensile forces on the fracture fragments

Closure

- Ensure adequate soft tissue coverage by closing the fascia directly over the plate
- Undue soft tissue tension should be avoided to reduce risk of wound breakdown
- Standard subcutaneous and skin closure is used
- The use of Steri-Strips should be avoided as these increase the chance of traction skin blisters
- No drainage is needed

Postoperative management

- In an uncomplicated olecranon fracture:
  - Apply a compressive bandage and start immediate mobilization
  - Alternatively, an extension splint with plaster backslab can be applied for 24–48 hours to reduce tension on wound
  - Commence early mobilization as soon as comfort allows
- In a complicated elbow fracture with ligament injury or reconstruction, further splinting or bracing may be required during rehabilitation

Early phase postoperative complications

- Superficial or deep infection
- Swelling
- Wound breakdown
- Blistering of the skin
- Ulnar neuropathy

Late phase postoperative complications

- Metalwork failure, e.g. backing-out of the screws
- Metalwork irritation necessitating removal
- Stiffness; however, up to 15° loss of terminal extension is to be expected
- Heterotopic ossification
- Ulnar nerve neuropathy, possibly due to fibrosis
- Malunion or nonunion
- Secondary osteoarthritis

Outpatient follow-up

- The patient is seen at 2 weeks for suture removal and radiographic assessment
- Further radiographic assessment is carried out at 3 and 6 months to ensure fracture union (**Figure 9.10**)

Implant removal

- It is not unusual for the metalwork to be removed due to its subcutaneous position causing local irritation or undue prominence

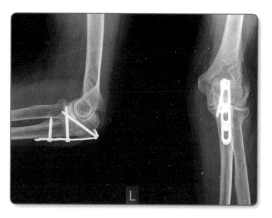

Figure 9.10 Postoperative check radiograph to ensure union. With permission of the MoRe Foundation.

- Plate removal is less common than removal of tension band cerclage wires
- This can be safely performed if the patient desires, after 6 months, and following radiographic assessment of union

- Patients should be preoperatively counseled about the need for this

Further reading

Den Hamer A, Heusinkveld M, Traa W, et al. Current techniques for management of transverse displaced olecranon fractures. Muscles Ligaments Tendons J 2015;5:129–140.

Wood T, Thomas K, Farrokhyar F, et al. A survey of current practices and preferences for internal fixation of displaced olecranon fractures. Can J Surg 2015; 58:250–256.

Fracture fixation for distal humeral intra-articular fractures

Indications

- Open reduction and internal fixation of distal humeral intra-articular fractures is a challenging procedure, and is indicated to reduce the risk of arthritis and avoid the need for an elbow replacement
- Elbow arthroplasty rather than fracture fixation can be considered as a primary procedure in a significantly comminuted fracture in an older patient with comorbidities

Preoperative assessment

Clinical assessment

- These are often high-energy injuries, and other injuries need to be excluded
- The soft tissue envelope needs to be assessed to identify an open fracture and determine immediate management
- The neurovascular status of the limb needs to be assessed and documented
- An above-elbow backslab will support the fracture while the patient is awaiting surgery

Imaging assessment

Radiographs

- Plain radiographs are useful but often underestimate the extent of the fracture

Computed tomography (CT)

- CT is useful in surgical planning
- Three-dimensional reconstructions of the CT images are helpful, but the software often fills in the space between bone pieces, which can hide the true extent of the fracture

Timing for surgery

- Open fractures should be fixed as soon as possible to reduce the risk of infection. If surgery cannot be performed immediately the wound should be cleaned and debrided, and an external fixator applied to stabilize the fracture
- Closed fractures should ideally be operated on within a week of the injury. Tissue dissection is harder if surgery is performed later

Surgical preparation

In a highly comminuted or complex fracture configuration, the surgeon should be prepared to convert to an elbow replacement if it is not possible to fix the fracture.

Surgical equipment

- The surgeon should use any elbow plating system available in their unit that they are comfortable employing
- It is important to ensure that all plate and screw options are available, including distal humeral and olecranon plates

Patient positioning

- The patient is positioned supine
- A bolster, sandbag, or bag of saline is placed under the shoulder blade of the injured arm to help to tilt the patient slightly towards the uninjured arm (**Figure 10.1**)
- The patient's shoulder needs to be positioned close to the edge of the operating table to allow intraoperative fluoroscopy
- A folded and taped pillow in a sterile Mayo bag (**Figures 10.2–10.4**) can be placed on the patient's chest to help to support the arm during surgery and free up the assistant
- During surgery, although the patient's forearm will rest on their chest, fluoroscopic images may be taken by positioning the elbow on the image intensifier by moving the shoulder (**Figures 10.5** and **10.6**)
- A high tourniquet

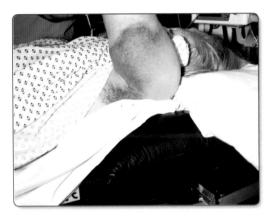

Figure 10.1 Place a sandbag or a large bag of saline under the ipsilateral shoulder.

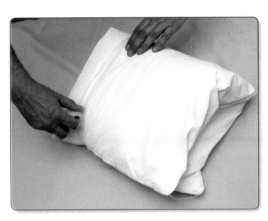

Figure 10.2 Fold a pillow and secure it with surgical tape.

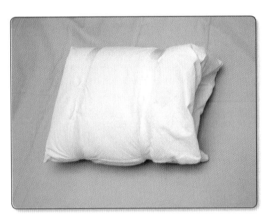

Figure 10.3 The folded and secured pillow.

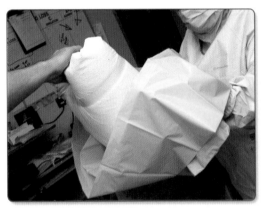

Figure 10.4 Place the pillow in a sterile Mayo bag.

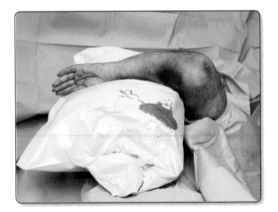

Figure 10.5 The arm resting on the wrapped pillow for surgery.

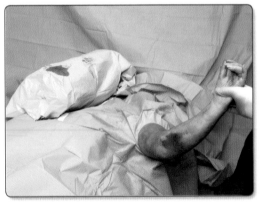

Figure 10.6 The arm can be extended for intraoperative fluoroscopy.

- Intravenous antibiotics according to local hospital policy and guidelines, administered before tourniquet inflation
- Chemical and mechanical prophylaxis for deep vein thrombosis according to local hospital policy and guidelines
- An image intensifier for intraoperative fluoroscopy

Surgical technique

Exposure

- Use a posterior midline incision, slightly curved round the olecranon (**Figure 10.7**)
- Identify the ulnar nerve and pass a sloop around the nerve to protect it (**Figure 10.8**)
- Consider releasing the tourniquet after the nerve has been identified and protected

There are several different approaches to the elbow:

1. **Olecranon osteotomy:** This is the best exposure for complex intra-articular fractures. It does, however, make conversion to a total elbow replacement challenging. This technique is described in more detail below
2. **Midline triceps split:** Although this proximally extensile approach gives a reasonable view for distal humeral extra-articular fractures, it does not provide adequate visualization for intra-articular fractures
3. **Triceps-reflecting approach:** After isolating the ulnar nerve, the triceps is released from the humerus and the medial and lateral intermuscular septa:
   - The triceps is then reflected medially or laterally, allowing exposure to the relevant column
   - The disadvantage of this technique is that it may only allow visualization of one column at a time, and the view of the entire articular surface is limited
   - This technique is useful for extra-articular fractures and simple intra-articular fractures
4. **The TRAP (triceps–anconeus reflecting pedicle) approach:** This approach involves

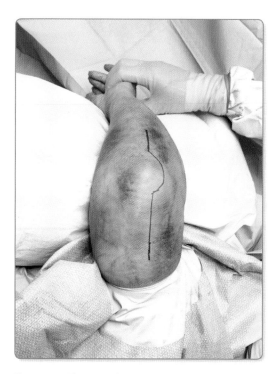

Figure 10.7 The surgical incision.

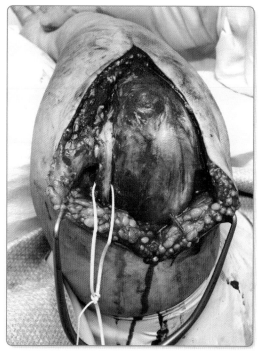

Figure 10.8 The ulnar nerve identified and protected with sloop.

combining the Bryan–Morrey and modified Kocher approaches to reflect the triceps in continuity with the anconeus:

- This approach partially detaches the triceps from the olecranon, which provides some additional exposure of the articular surface
- There is a risk of detaching the collateral ligaments, which can lead to instability

Although the articular surface exposure is not as good as with the olecranon osteotomy, it is easy to convert to a total elbow replacement if necessary.

Olecranon osteotomy technique

- After identifying and protecting the ulnar nerve, release the triceps medially and laterally from the intermuscular septa
- Expose either side of the proximal olecranon

- Apply an olecranon plate to the bone prior to the osteotomy to help olecranon reduction and plate alignment at the end of the operation (**Figure 10.9**)
- After applying the plate, drill and insert two screws proximally and two distally. Inserting two screws at either end will provide rotational control of the fracture when reducing the osteotomy. Additional screws will also be required at the end of the procedure. Also drill the hole for the long intramedullary screw but do not insert the screw
- Remove the screws and plate prior to the osteotomy
- The articular surface of the ulna has a 'bare area' devoid of cartilage that lies in the middle

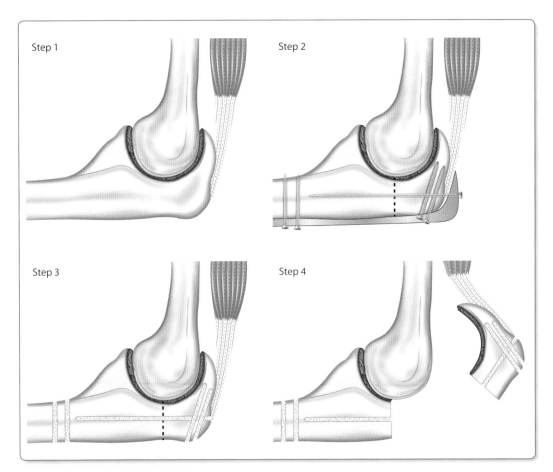

Figure 10.9 Apply an olecranon plate to the bone prior to the osteotomy to help olecranon reduction and plate alignment at the end of the operation. Drill, insert and then remove the shorter screws. Drill the hole for the long screw but do not insert it at this stage. Long screw shown for illustrative purposes only.

of the olecranon articular area. This is the site of the olecranon osteotomy (**Figure 10.10**)
- Intraoperative fluoroscopy can be used to identify the osteotomy site
- The osteotomy can be initiated with a saw blade irrigated with saline to avoid thermal necrosis of the bone, and completed with an osteotome
- The olecranon is then reflected with the triceps to expose the fracture

Fracture reduction
- The basic principle is to restore the articular surface and then secure the reconstructed articular area to the remaining bone (**Figure 10.11**)
- Fracture reduction is the most important and most difficult part of the surgical procedure
- Temporarily stabilize the reduction with Kirschner wires
- Once the bone is temporarily stable, apply the plate and screws
- The Mayo clinic has described surgical objectives for a stable fixation of these fractures:
  - Screws in the distal articular segment should be of adequate number and as long as possible
  - These screws should pass through a plate and engage a fragment on the opposite side that is also fixed to a plate
  - Each screw should engage as many articular fragments as possible

- The screws should lock together by interdigitation, thereby creating a fixed-angle construct linking the columns
  - Plates used for fixation should achieve compression at the supracondylar level for both columns. The plates must be strong and stiff to resist breaking or bending before fracture union
- Modern precontoured plates are available for this type of fracture, but these may need to be contoured further by the surgeon to fit the anatomy of the individual patient

Two plate options are available (**Figure 10.12**):
1. Parallel plates applied to the medial and lateral aspects of the humerus
2. 90–90 plates, i.e. plates at 90° to each other, applied to the medial and posterior aspects of the humerus, i.e. plates at 90° to each other. The distal screws in the radial side of the articular segment are unicortical to avoid joint protrusion, and therefore provide less stable fixation. This may be appropriate for simple extra-articular fractures, but with intra-articular fractures an additional 'lateral support' plate may be needed that allows screws to be passed across the fracture from lateral to medial (**Figure 10.12**)

Possible perioperative complications
- Infection
- Neurovascular injury

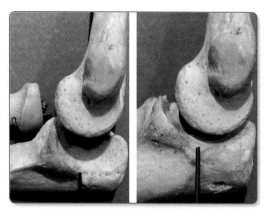

Figure 10.10 Bare area on the olecranon shown by red pointer.

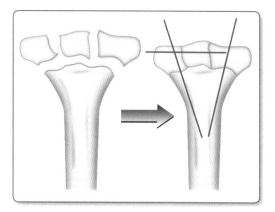

Figure 10.11 Reduce the fracture and stabilize it with Kirschner wires.

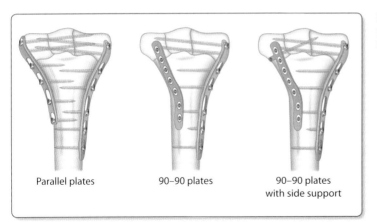

Figure 10.12 Parallel plates, 90–90 plates, and 90–90 plates with lateral support.

Parallel plates   90–90 plates   90–90 plates
                                               with side support

- Wound breakdown
- Failure of fixation
- Stiffness

Closure

- After fracture fixation, the olecranon is reduced
- The olecranon plate can be used as a reduction tool (**Figure 10.13**):
  - Insert the locking guide into the hole at end of the plate for the long intramedullary screw
  - Detach the drill bit from the drill and slide it into a drill guide that is already attached to the plate
  - Apply the plate to the proximal olecranon fragment and slide the drill through the hole in the bone so that the tip is just protruding at the osteotomy site
  - The tip of the drill can then be passed into the predrilled intramedullary hole in the distal ulnar fragment
  - Once the ulnar is reduced, insert screws into the plate holes. Additional screws may be needed
  - After the plate is secure, remove the drill bit and locking guide. Finally, measure and insert the intramedullary screw
- Check the ulnar nerve and transpose it anteriorly unless it is lying in a position where it will not be irritated by the metalwork
- Check the integrity of the collateral ligaments prior to closing the fat and skin

Postoperative management

- Apply a bulky dressing, backslab, and sling
- If the skin quality and fixation are satisfactory, consider providing the patient with a removable resting sling or cast, and commence early mobilization
- If there are concerns about the skin quality, inspect the wound before discharge and immobilize it until the 10–14-day clinic review

Outpatient follow-up

- Review in the clinic at 10–14 days for a wound check and radiograph
- If the review is satisfactory and the fracture fixation was stable intraoperatively, commence gentle range of motion exercises
- If there are any concerns regarding fracture fixation or patient compliance, consider a further short period of immobilization. The patient and surgeon should be aware that this can lead to stiffness that may require additional treatment later
- By 6 weeks the bone should be strong enough to commence strengthening and range of motion exercises. If the elbow is very stiff at 6 weeks, consider a gentle examination or manipulation under anesthesia to help with movement

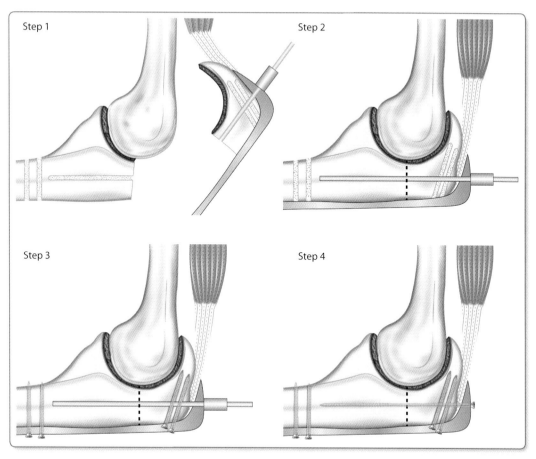

Step 1

Step 2

Step 3

Step 4

Figure 10.13 Closure of the osteotomy. The locking guide has been placed into the plate hole and the unmounted drill bit passed through it into the proximal olecranon. The tip of drill then slides into the previously drilled intramedullary hole in the distal ulnar segment to help the reduction.

Further reading

Wang AA, Mara M, Hutchinson DT. The proximal ulna: an anatomic study with relevance to olecranon osteotomy and fracture fixation. J Shoulder Elbow Surg 2003; 12:293–296.

Sanchez-Sotelo J, Torchia ME, O'Driscoll SW. Complex distal humeral fractures: internal fixation with a principle-based parallel-plate technique. Surgical technique. J Bone Joint Surg Am 2008; 90:31–46.

Flexible intramedullary nailing for pediatric supracondylar humeral fracture

Indications

- Flexible intramedullary nailing (FIN) in pediatric supracondylar humeral fractures can be used for Gartland type III fractures, i.e. when there is both anterior and posterior cortical disruption associated with a displacement
- One of the main advantages of this technique is the management of comminuted fractures

Preoperative assessment

Clinical assessment

Rigorous initial examination is crucial to detect associated soft tissues injuries:

- Nerve injury in supracondylar fractures can occur in 5–10% of cases. Motor and sensory examination should be performed for the three main upper limb nerves: median, ulnar, and radial. Injury to the anterior interosseous nerve (a branch of the median nerve) is classically described with these fractures and is indicated by an inability to bend the interphalangeal joint of the thumb
- Vascular injury must be assessed by checking the radial and ulnar pulses, and a vascular opinion sought if there are any concerns. As an important vascular collateral blood supply exists in children, a humeral artery injury can exist without causing distal ischemia, i.e. the 'pink pulseless hand'. If this persists after fracture reduction, a vascular opinion is mandatory
- Open fracture necessitates prophylactic antibiotic treatment in accordance with local hospital policy and guidelines. The authors recommend antibiotics for 3 days

Imaging assessment

- Standard anteroposterior and lateral radiographs of the elbow are sufficient to diagnose supracondylar fractures (**Figure 11.1**)
- Around 10% of cases have an associated fracture, most commonly a distal radius fracture. The authors recommend routine radiographs of the forearm in all cases
- For a pink, pulseless hand, intraoperative arteriography should be performed by the vascular surgeon if the pulse does not return after fracture reduction
- In cases of arterial injury, a vascular repair should be performed after fracture stabilization

Timing for surgery

- Supracondylar fractures are surgical emergencies and surgery must be performed in the first 24 hours. If surgery is delayed by

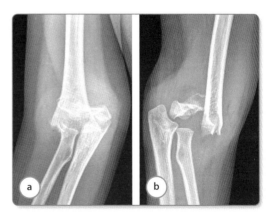

Figure 11.1 Anteroposterior (a) and lateral (b) radiographs of the elbow, showing a Gartland type III supracondylar humeral fracture with a posteromedial displacement.

48 hours, open reduction may be necessary as percutaneous reduction may not be possible
- In cases of neurovascular injury, surgery should be performed urgently within 6 hours

Surgical preparation

Surgical equipment

The equipment required for FIN is shown in **Figure 11.2** and includes:

- A surgical awl
- A T-handle
- A hammer
- Intramedullary nails:
  - The ideal nail diameter is between 1.5 and 2.0 mm depending on the age of the child. If intramedullary nails are not available, FIN is still possible using long Kirschner wires by cutting the sharp end of the wires
  - Bending the nails is a crucial step in the FIN technique. Nails must be bent in the distal third to facilitate placement in the medial and lateral columns of the distal humeral metaphysis (**Figure 11.3**)
  - The distal extremity needs to be manipulated to avoid impingement of the fracture cortex when introducing the nails
- A fluoroscopic imaging system

Of note, an inflatable tourniquet is not used.

Equipment positioning

The image intensifier is placed parallel to the operating table on the side of the injured limb

Patient positioning

- The patient is positioned supine with the injured limb on a radiolucent arm table. The patient must be carefully positioned near the edge of the table to facilitate fluoroscopic imaging

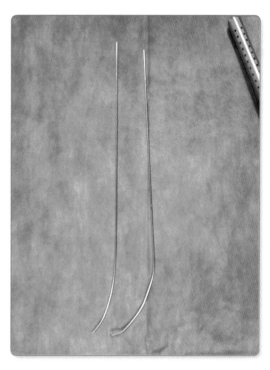

Figure 11.3 Long Kirschner wires used for flexible intramedullary nailing. The nails or wires must be bent at the distal third.

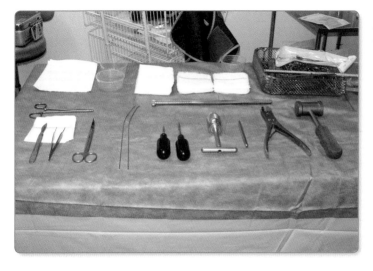

Figure 11.2 Instrumentation table with the instruments needed for flexible intramedullary nailing.

- A pelvic support is sometimes needed to provide additional support on the operating table
- Fracture reduction is performed at this stage to ensure that an open reduction is not needed
- Then the entire upper limb is prepared and draped for surgery

Further preparation

As a standard orthopaedic surgical procedure with internal osteosynthesis, intraoperative prophylactic antibiotic treatment is administered in accordance with local hospital policy and guidelines.

Surgical technique

Exposure

- A 1 cm skin incision is made on the lateral aspect of the arm at the deltoid tuberosity. The soft tissues down to bone are dissected with the scissors pointing distally (**Figure 11.4**)

Introduction of the nails

- An awl is inserted into the wound. The surgeon must feel the anterior and posterior cortex to ensure the correct nail entry point. The lateral cortex of the humeral shaft is trephined at the distal end of the skin incision in a distal direction (**Figure 11.5**)
- Nails are then introduced into the medullary canal using a T-handle with gentle rotatory movements

- The first nail is advanced to just proximal of the fracture site in the medial column. The distal end of the nail must be directed medially
- The second nail is advanced through the humeral shaft, but the T-handle is turned 180° to push the nail into the lateral column. The distal end of the nail must be directed laterally
- The two nails must sit just proximal to the fracture site and point in opposite directions (**Figure 11.6**)

Fracture reduction

- Reduction is performed by external manipulation
- A longitudinal traction is applied to the upper limb and countertraction to the forearm. Fracture disimpaction is confirmed under fluoroscopic control
- Based on the initial displacement, the forearm is placed in either pronation or supination to maintain rotational stability
- The elbow is flexed with one hand on the forearm, while the other hand pushes the olecranon forward (**Figure 11.7**)
- Anteroposterior and lateral fluoroscopic images ensure satisfactory fracture reduction

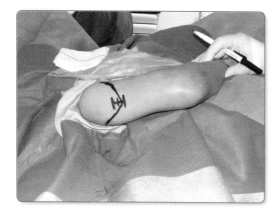

Figure 11.4 The skin incision must be performed at the deltoid tuberosity. Dissection is then carried out in a distal direction.

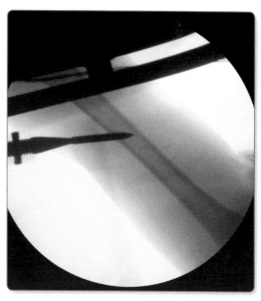

Figure 11.5 Fluoroscopic image of the entry point of the nail in the humeral shaft. The awl is introduced pointing distally.

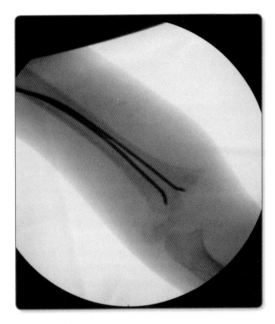

Figure 11.6 Fluoroscopic image prior to fracture reduction, showing the nails advanced to just above the fracture site in the lateral and medial columns.

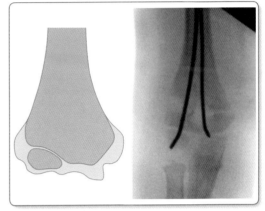

Figure 11.8 Fluoroscopic image demonstrating the final nail positions. In view of the mostly cartilaginous distal humerus in children, the nails must protrude beyond the bony margins seen on fluoroscopy.

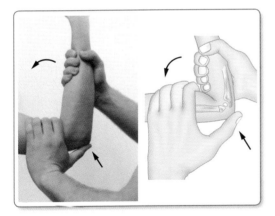

Figure 11.7 The reduction maneuver with the elbow flexed with one hand on the forearm, while the other hand pushes the olecranon forward.

Final osteosynthesis

- Crossing the fracture site with the nails is the key step in this technique
- While the surgeon maintains the reduction, an assistant advances the nails past the fracture site with a hammer

- The first nail is advanced into the lateral column until it reaches the capitellum. It must be directed anterolaterally
- The second nail is advanced into the medial column until it reaches the trochlea. It must be directed medially
- As most of the distal humerus is cartilaginous in children, the nails must protrude beyond the bony margins seen on fluoroscopy in order to ensure adequate stability (**Figure 11.8**)

End of procedure

- Final fluoroscopic images at the extremes of flexion and extension are saved to confirm fracture stability
- The nails are then cut at the proximal end at 1 cm from the entry point and bent to avoid soft tissue irritation

Possible perioperative complications

- Inability to achieve perfect reduction: if external manipulation fails to achieve perfect reduction, further reduction can be attempted

by using the T-handle to rotate the nails in the distal fragment. If this fails, open reduction with Kirschner wire stabilization can be considered
- Misplacement of the nails: a third nail can be inserted while reduction is maintained by the earlier two nails. Once the third nail is adequately positioned, the misplaced nail can be removed or left in situ (**Figure 11.9**)

Closure

- The wound is closed in two layers
- The upper limb is placed in a brachio-antebrachial splint for the first 10 days to reduce postoperative pain

Postoperative management

- Postoperatively, the child must be observed for 24–48 hours for compartment syndrome

- Standard postoperative anteroposterior and lateral radiographs are performed before discharge (**Figure 11.10**)
- The splint is removed after 10 days and the elbow allowed to move freely
- Physiotherapy is contraindicated in children because of the risk of periarticular ectopic ossification
- A full range of motion is generally achieved after 6–12 months

Implant removal

- Bone healing is generally achieved 4–6 weeks postoperatively
- Metalwork removal can be performed 2–3 months postoperatively
- Metalwork removal is performed under general anesthesia through the same skin incision, as a day-case procedure
- No immobilization is required after metalwork removal

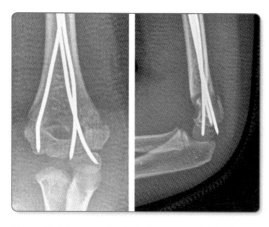

Figure 11.9 In cases of nail misplacement, a third nail can be inserted while reduction is maintained by the earlier two nails. Once the third nail is adequately positioned, the misplaced nail can be removed or left in situ.

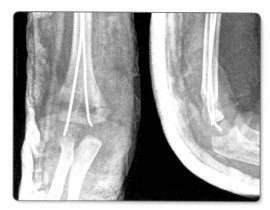

Figure 11.10 Postoperative radiographs showing restored distal humerus anteversion. The upper limb is placed in a long arm splint for the first few postoperative days.

Further reading

Lagrange J, Rigault P. Fractures supracondyliennes. Rev Chir Orthop 1962; 48:337–414.

Journeau P, Annocaro F. Supracondylar humeral fracture. In: Lascombes P, Annocaro F, Barbary S, et al. (eds), Flexible intramedullary nailing in children: the Nancy University manual. Berlin: Springer-Verlag, 2010: 115–135.

Ligier JN, Metaizeau JP, Prevot J. Closed flexible medullary nailing in pediatric traumatology. Chir Pediatr 1983; 24:383–385.

Prevot J, Lascombes P, Métaizeau JP, Blanquart D. Supracondylar fractures of the humerus in children: treatment by downward nailing. Rev Chir Orthop Réparatrice Appar Mot 1990; 76:191–197.

Acute ligamentous repair following elbow dislocation

Indications

Surgery is indicated in elbow dislocations that:

- Are associated with concomitant displaced fractures involving the radial head, coronoid, olecranon, or epicondyle
- Remain unstable in more than 30° of flexion and pronation after reduction
- Re-dislocate with a passive range of motion or during plaster immobilization

The surgical management of unstable simple dislocations, i.e. dislocations without associated fractures, involves the repair or reconstruction of the lateral ulnar collateral ligament (LUCL) and/or medial collateral ligament (MCL)

Preoperative assessment

Clinical assessment

- Patients with acute elbow dislocation tend to present with pain, soft tissue swelling, and a deformed elbow
- A neurovascular examination of the upper extremity should always be performed
- The wrist and shoulder joints should be carefully examined to rule out concomitant upper extremity injuries. The distal radioulnar joint and forearm interosseous membrane should always be examined for tenderness and instability to rule out any associated injuries
- Following the successful reduction of an acute elbow dislocation, the range of motion and stability of the elbow are assessed. It is important to assess the stability of the elbow in a position of near-full or full extension as the elbow is generally stable at 90° or more of flexion

Imaging assessment

Radiographs

- Anteroposterior and lateral radiographs are normally sufficient to diagnose the dislocation

and determine the direction of forearm displacement
- The radiographs should be carefully assessed to identify any associated fractures
- Postreduction radiographs are assessed for joint widening, irregularity, and malalignment, which may indicate posterolateral rotatory instability or the interposition of soft tissue or osteochondral fragments

Computed tomography (CT)

- If there is any doubt as to the radiographic findings, CT should be performed after reduction of the dislocation

Timing for surgery

- Surgery should be performed as soon as possible if the surgical indications above have been met

Surgical preparation

Repair of the lateral ligament complex will normally restore elbow stability, and it is rarely necessary to address the MCL.

Surgical equipment

- Heavy nonabsorbable no. 5 sutures
- High speed burr with 2 mm burr
- 5.5 mm nonabsorbable or absorbable anchors
- Sometimes a hinge external fixator may be required

Equipment positioning

- C-arm radiographic equipment is positioned at the head of the patient
- No other equipment is needed

Patient positioning

- Patients are positioned supine with the arm on a radiolucent hand table
- The forearm is kept in pronation to increase the distance between the lateral approach and the posterior interosseous nerve

Further preparation

- A tourniquet is placed on the proximal part of the arm

Surgical technique

Exposure

- A lateral incision is made along the lateral humeral column, extending down to the lateral aspect of the ulna
- After the skin incision and subcutaneous dissection, the lateral epicondyle is explored
- The lateral extensor origin may have avulsed from the lateral epicondyle, exposing the joint (**Figure 12.1**)
- If the extensor origin is intact, Kocher's interval is opened between the extensor carpi ulnaris and the anconeus to visualize the LUCL (**Figure 12.2**)
- A band of fat tissue usually identifies the limits of Kocher's interval
- The anterior capsule is opened laterally and the joint is entered. The radial head and coronoid process are inspected. If there are fractures, fixation or replacement is performed as described in Chapters 10 and 11

LUCL repair

- The origin of the LUCL is identified on the deep surface of the anterior capsule
- A running no. 5 nonabsorbable Krackow locking suture is placed on the anterior half of the capsulo-ligamentous fibers from proximal to distal, and then from distal to proximal, turning at the ulnar supinator crest (**Figure 12.3**)

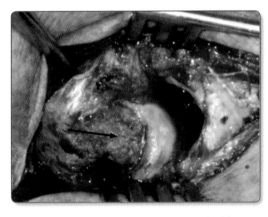

Figure 12.1 The lateral extensor origin has avulsed from the lateral epicondyle, exposing the joint.

Figure 12.2 If the extensor origin is intact, Kocher's interval is opened between the extensor carpi ulnaris and the anconeus to visualize the lateral ulnar collateral ligament.

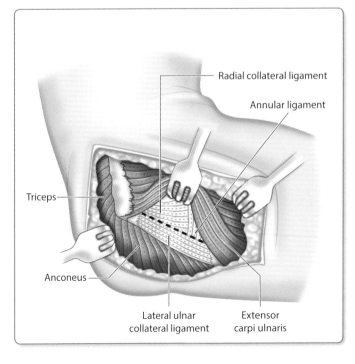

Radial collateral ligament

Annular ligament

Triceps

Anconeus

Lateral ulnar collateral ligament

Extensor carpi ulnaris

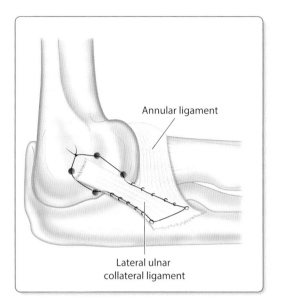

Figure 12.3 A running Krackow locking suture is placed on the anterior half of the capsulo-ligamentous fibers from proximal to distal, and then from distal to proximal, turning at the ulnar supinator crest.

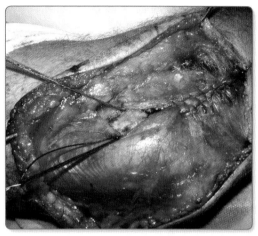

Figure 12.4 The limbs of the running suture are passed through the humeral tunnels.

- A second suture is placed in the same fashion on the posterior half of the capsulo-ligamentous fibers. These sutures may be passed through the overlying common extensor–supinator fibers to augment the repair
- The isometric origin on the humerus is then identified at the center of the capitellum. Confirmation of the isometric point is made by clamping the two limbs of the running suture at the point of isometry, and then flexing and extending the elbow
- A 2.0 mm burr is used to make a humeral bone tunnel. It is important to make the isometric point the most anterior aspect of the bone tunnel, and not the center of the tunnel, as any translation can result in a lax LUCL repair in extension
- Two 'exit' tunnels, one anterior and one posterior to the lateral column, are then made with a 2.0 mm burr. These are connected to the distal humeral tunnel at the isometric point in a Y-configuration
- The limbs of the running suture are passed through the humeral tunnels (**Figure 12.4**)
- The joint is concentrically reduced under fluoroscopic imaging, and the LUCL repair

sutures tied with the elbow flexed 45° and the forearm in pronation
- The stability of the elbow is assessed through an arc of motion, looking for posterior displacement of the radial head relative to the capitellum in extension, which suggests either a lax LUCL or a nonisometric repair
- If the elbow is stable through an arc of motion, the extensor origin is repaired with interrupted, heavy no. 0 nonabsorbable sutures, and the skin is closed in layers

MCL repair

- If the elbow remains unstable after the LUCL repair, acute avulsion of the MCL and the flexor origin should be suspected and will need to be repaired
- An acute injury rarely requires a reconstruction with a graft, and it is normally possible to repair the MCL and flexor origin with sutures
- When exposing the medial side of the joint, the ulnar nerve must be identified and protected
- In most cases, the flexor origin will have avulsed from the medial epicondyle, and the underlying disrupted MCL will be easily visualized

- The MCL is mobilized and repaired by placing Bunnell-type nonabsorbable sutures through the ligament and then passing the suture ends through drill holes in the medial epicondyle
- The sutures are securely tied over the medial epicondyle
- The flexor mass is then securely repaired with further drill holes through the bone

Hinged external fixation

- External fixation can be used in rare cases if bony and ligamentous stability cannot be achieved and the elbow re-dislocates in a well-fitting cast or splint. This is more likely to be the case with concomitant fractures, especially a comminuted coronoid fracture not amenable to plate or screw fixation
- Hinged external fixators are positioned so that the center of rotation lies at the center of the capitellum laterally and just anteroinferior to the medial epicondyle at the center of the trochlea medially
- The pins are placed in line with the center of rotation and parallel to the joint surface. The position is confirmed by fluoroscopy
- The external fixator rod is aligned with the anterior humeral cortex
- The interepicondylar width defines a safe location for placement of the proximal humeral pin, as shown in **Figure 12.5**
- Once the external fixator has been applied (**Figure 12.6**), the elbow is taken through an arc of motion to ensure reduction is maintained. Fixators are usually used for 4–6 weeks

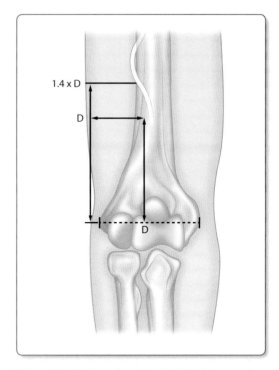

Figure 12.5 The interepicondylar width (D) defines a safe location for placement of the proximal humeral pin.

Possible perioperative complications

- When inserting external fixator pins, care must be taken to avoid injuring the radial nerve proximally with the proximal pin, and distally around the supinator muscle and the radial neck
- A safe zone must be used proximally when positioning the humeral pins
- The forearm must be held pronated to increase the distance between the lateral approach and the posterior interosseus nerve

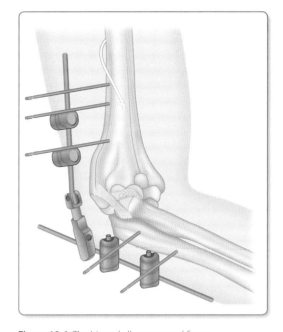

Figure 12.6 The hinged elbow external fixator.

Closure

- Close the space between the tendons with an absorbable suture
- A surgical drain is often required
- Close subcutaneous and skin layers in a standard fashion
- Simple dressing

Postoperative management

- After operative stabilization without external fixation, the elbow is splinted in 90° flexion with the forearm in pronation for 2 weeks to allow wound healing
- A hinged orthosis is applied after 2 weeks with the forearm in pronation and allowing a range of motion from 30° to full flexion

- At 6 weeks the splint is removed and a full range of motion is allowed. Flexion–extension exercises are performed with the forearm in pronation, and pronation–supination exercises are performed with the elbow in 90° of flexion

Outpatient follow-up

- A 2-week outpatient clinic review is scheduled for wound inspection and a change of splint
- The 6-week review is for removal of the splint and a physiotherapy review
- The patient is then reviewed 3-monthly until they have regained a full range of movement and resumed normal activities

Further reading

Ahmad CS, ElAttrache NS. Treatment of medial ulnar collateral ligament injuries in athletes. In: Morrey BF (ed.), Master techniques in orthopaedic surgery: the elbow, 3rd edn. Philadelphia: Wolters Kluwer, 2015; 347–362.

Morrey BF, Sanchez-Sotelo J. Surgical repair and reconstruction of the lateral ulnar collateral ligament. In: Morrey BF (ed.), Master techniques in orthopaedic surgery: the elbow, 3rd edn. Philadelphia: Wolters Kluwer, 2015;375–387.

Morrey BF. Articulated external fixators. In: Morrey BF (ed.), Master techniques in orthopaedic surgery: the elbow, 3rd edn. Philadelphia: Wolters Kluwer, 2015; 157–170.

Arthroscopic debridement for posteromedial impingement

Indications

- Athletes with posteromedial elbow pain on elbow extension
- Athletes with valgus extension overload and posteromedial elbow pain

Preoperative assessment

Clinical assessment

- Posteromedial elbow pain is typically seen in young athletes
- Patients will typically complain of pain on full elbow extension and exacerbated by activity
- Activities requiring forceful full extension such a pitching, bowling, or sparring are particularly aggravating
- On examination the patient may have an elbow effusion, suggested by filling of the lateral soft spot and limited extension
- Marked synovitis may be palpable in the posteromedial recess
- Pushing the elbow into full extension while palpating the posteromedial gutter may reproduce the pain
- The medial collateral ligament of the elbow should be examined as posteromedial impingement may be a sign of valgus extension overload of the elbow
- The ulnar nerve should be clinically examined and the findings documented. If there is evidence of pre-existing nerve entrapment, a decompression should be performed with the elbow arthroscopy

Imaging assessment

Radiographs

- Plain radiographs can demonstrate osteophytes on the medial aspect of the olecranon and posteromedial aspect of the trochlea, but these can be difficult to identify

- Loose bodies may also be present on plain radiographs

Magnetic resonance imaging (MRI)

- MRI is the investigation of choice. This may show increased signal within the bone on either side of the posteromedial gutter on T2-weighted images
- Synovitis may be visible
- Osteophytes can be identified, and occasionally a fracture of a posteromedial osteophyte may be seen
- In valgus extension overload, there may be visible thinning of the cartilage in the posteromedial articulation of the ulnohumeral joint

Timing for surgery

- Surgical timing is likely to be dictated by the demands of the athlete. Unless they are unable to continue with their sporting activities due to their symptoms, they may choose to plan surgery for the end of a season
- In severe cases, surgery may be more urgent to hasten a return to sporting activities
- Intra-articular local steroid injections may ameliorate acute symptoms to allow a return to sporting activities, with a planned procedure at a later, more convenient time

Surgical preparation

Surgical equipment

- A 4 mm arthroscope with forward-flowing cannula
- A fluid management system
- Arthroscopic tools including an arthroscopic shaver
- Both soft tissue and bone-cutting shaver blades
- Arthroscopic retractors to minimize the risk of injury to the ulnar nerve, and to enhance the

arthroscopic visualization of the posteromedial recess

Equipment positioning

- The arthroscopic stack is positioned behind the laterally positioned patient and opposite the surgeon
- The fluid management settings should be clearly visible to the surgeon
- If foot pedals are to be used, these should be placed where the surgeon can operate them comfortably
- A Mayo stand is positioned over the patient's shoulder to provide a flat surface for the surgical instruments

Patient positioning

- The patient is placed in the lateral decubitus position and the surgeon stands in front of them
- The prone position can also be used
- The lateral positioning is facilitated by the use of a positioning suction beanbag, or pelvic supports and Trimano limb holder (Maquet) with elbow attachment (Arthrex) (**Figure 13.1**)
- A high upper arm tourniquet is applied high enough to allow portal placement. It may be necessary to use a narrow tourniquet

Further preparation

- 20 mL of 7.5% ropivacaine should be instilled into the elbow joint using a hypodermic needle placed at the site of the posterior midline

portal and directed towards the olecranon fossa (**Figure 13.2**)

Surgical technique

Exposure

- Routine elbow arthroscopy is performed with visualization of all three compartments: posterior, anterior, and lateral
- For evaluation of the posteromedial recess, it is best to initially use the posterior midline portal to view the recess (**Figure 13.3**)
- Debridement of the posteromedial recess is best performed using a 3.5 mm soft tissue resector through the posterior midline portal

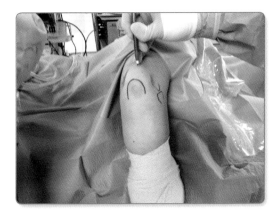

Figure 13.2   Initial posterior midline portal for elbow arthroscopy.

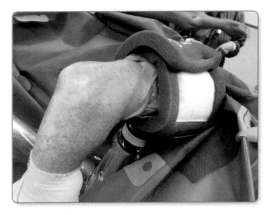

Figure 13.1   Positioning for elbow arthroscopy.

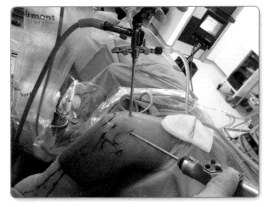

Figure 13.3   A posterior midline viewing portal and a posterolateral working portal.

while the camera is inserted through the posterolateral portal (**Figure 13.4**). This affords better and safer access for removal of synovitis without risk of iatrogenic ulnar nerve injury

- **Figure 13.5** shows a 'loose body' attached to the synovial lining that is removed
- A hooded shaver should be used with the hood always directed towards the ulnar nerve
- **Figures 13.6** and **13.7** show arthroscopic views demonstrating debridement for posteromedial impingement
- Arthroscopic retractors significantly improve joint visualization and safety of the procedure

Possible perioperative complications

- The greatest risk is of injury to the ulnar nerve, which lies in close proximity to the posteromedial gutter. In experienced hands the risk of nerve injury is less than 1%, but higher rates have been reported and probably

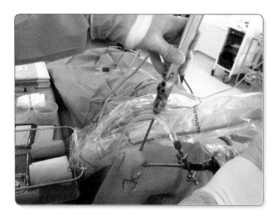

Figure 13.4 An alternative setup with a posterolateral viewing portal and a posterior midline working portal.

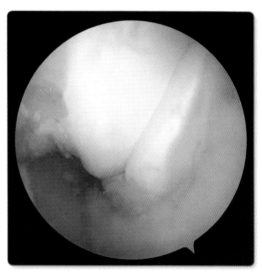

Figure 13.6 An arthroscopic view demonstrating debridement for posteromedial impingement.

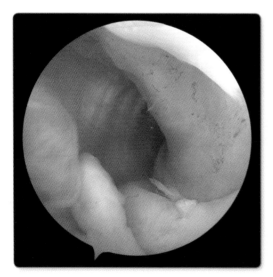

Figure 13.5 A 'loose body' attached to the synovial lining in posteromedial impingement.

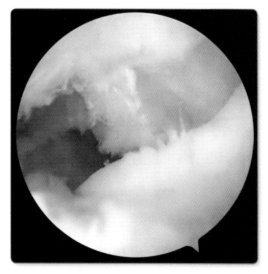

Figure 13.7 An arthroscopic view of the posteromedial recess with the elbow in extension after arthroscopic debridement.

reflect a learning curve for this procedure. Most lesions are neurapraxias
- Bleeding from portal sites and hematomas are common but rarely a serious complication
- Sinus formation at the portal sites has been reported following elbow arthroscopy but is rare even without formal suture closure
- The patient should be warned of the risk of recurrence. If the primary pathology is of injury or attenuation of the medial collateral ligament of the elbow due to valgus extension overload, recurrence is inevitable unless this is also addressed

Closure

- Small portal wounds are closed with Steri-Strips and a waterproof dressing
- Larger wounds, such as those used for ulnar nerve decompression, may require subcuticular suture closure
- A wool and crepe bandage is applied
- A sling is provided for comfort

Further reading

Cohen SB, Valko C, Zoga A, et al. Posteromedial elbow impingement: magnetic resonance imaging findings in overhead throwing athletes and results of arthroscopic treatment. Arthroscopy 2011; 27:1364–1370.

Postoperative management

- In the acute postoperative phase, analgesia and edema control with elevation and cryotherapy can enhance recovery
- The bandage should be removed at 48 hours to encourage active movement, and the sling discarded as soon as comfort allows
- An active range of movement with open- and closed-chain exercises should be encouraged from the 1st postoperative week
- Sport-specific training can commence as soon as a full pain-free active range of movement is achieved

Outpatient follow-up

- The patient is reviewed at 2 weeks postoperatively, and if satisfactory progress has been made, a sport-specific rehabilitation regimen can commence
- At the final 6-week follow-up, patients should have returned to their pre-injury sporting activities

Treatment of chronic posterolateral instability of the elbow

Indications

- Surgery is indicated for chronic symptomatic posterolateral (rotatory) instability of the elbow
- Posterolateral rotatory instability is related to lateral collateral ligament (LCL) attenuation, most often following elbow dislocations, or from iatrogenic injury during a lateral approach during surgery

Preoperative assessment

Clinical assessment

Patient history

- Symptoms and clinical signs in LCL insufficiency vary depending on the severity of the instability
- Most commonly, patients complain of lateral elbow pain with clicking, snapping, or locking, particularly when the elbow is actively extended with the forearm supinated. In rare cases of LCL insufficiency, recurrent frank elbow dislocations can occur
- Daily activities such as pushing to stand up from a chair or lifting objects in supination induce symptoms. In some patients these activities are even impossible to perform due to 'apprehension'

Physical examination

- In patients with symptoms suggestive of LCL insufficiency, identification of post-traumatic deformities such as cubitus varus or valgus and the location of previous skin incisions are important. Skin incisions on the lateral side may be associated with ligamentous injury
- Several physical examination maneuvers are used to test the LCL:
  - The pivot shift maneuver described by O'Driscoll involves applying a valgus, supinatory, and axial load force to the elbow (**Figure 14.1**). As the elbow is extended,

the radial head and ulna sublux from the humerus. During flexion the elbow relocates (**Figure 14.2**). However, in the majority of patients this pivot shift is hard to elicit without anesthesia, although most patients report painful apprehension at 30–50° of flexion
  - Alternatively the 'push–up' test described by Regan can be used to assess posterolateral instability. The patient is asked to push their bodyweight out of an armchair while

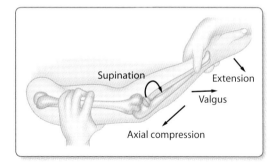

Figure 14.1 The pivot shift maneuver with a valgus, supinatory, and axial load force applied to the elbow. As the elbow is extended, the radial head and ulna sublux from the humerus.

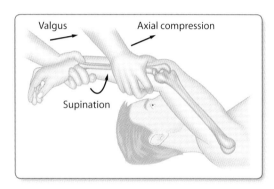

Figure 14.2 As the elbow is flexed, the joint relocates.

keeping the forearms in supination and the shoulders abducted. If the patient has PLRI, it is impossible to perform this test since extension of the elbow results in subluxation of the radiocapitellar joint

- A similar test is the 'table top' test. The patient reports apprehension when asked to perform a press-up with the elbow pointing laterally. Pain and apprehension occur as the elbow reaches approximately 40° of flexion, and these symptoms improve or resolve when the test is repeated with the examiner using their thumb to push over the radial head, preventing posterior subluxation

- The posterolateral rotator drawer test can also be used to demonstrate posterolateral subluxation of the proximal radius and ulna with forced supination. For this test, the patient is positioned supine with the shoulder locked in maximal internal rotation. Forced supination of the forearm in 45° of flexion induces excessive posterolateral movement, which in severe cases results in subluxation of the elbow joint (**Figure 14.3**). As with the pivot shift test, the drawer test is hard to elicit without anesthesia, although apprehension is reported

Imaging assessment

Plain radiographs

Most patients with isolated LCL insufficiency present with normal plain radiographs. Most of the time, however, radiographs are helpful to delineate associated pathology, including post-traumatic changes at the radial head or coronoid, or varus malalignment of the distal humerus

Stress radiographs and fluoroscopy

- The forearm is placed in full supination and a varus load is applied to determine the amount of lateral joint line opening. More than 2 mm of opening usually indicates LCL insufficiency
- Posterolateral rotatory instability is best demonstrated on lateral views. With forced supination and valgus, the radius and ulna are subluxed posteriorly so that the center of the radial head no longer aligns with the center of the capitellum, and there is asymmetry and widening of the ulnohumeral joint

Magnetic resonance imaging (MRI) with arthrogram

- The different components of the LCL complex may be visualized using MRI. Negative findings on MRI do not exclude the diagnosis of posterolateral rotatory instability
- Intra-articular contrast injection can increase the likelihood that MRI will diagnose LCL attenuations or tears

Timing for surgery

- Surgery takes place following medical evaluation of the patient

Surgical preparation

Surgical equipment

- Heavy nonabsorbable no. 2 and no. 5 sutures
- High speed burr with 2 mm and 4 mm burr
- Sometimes a hinge external fixator may be required

Equipment positioning

- C-arm radiographic equipment is positioned at the head of the patient
- The forearm is prepared to take a palmaris longus tendon graft
- No other equipment is needed

Patient positioning

- Patients are positioned supine with the arm on a radiolucent hand table

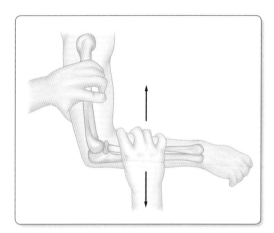

Figure 14.3 The posterolateral rotator drawer test where forced supination of the forearm in 45° of flexion induces excessive posterolateral movement.

- The forearm is kept in pronation to increase the distance between the lateral approach and the posterior interosseous nerve

Further preparation

- A high tourniquet is placed on the upper arm

Surgical technique

Exposure

- A lateral approach is usually performed along the lateral column, extending down to the lateral aspect of the ulna
- After skin incision and dissection of the subcutaneous layers, the lateral epicondyle is explored
- Kocher's interval is opened between the extensor carpi ulnaris and the anconeus
- A band of fat tissue usually identifies the limits of Kocher's interval
- The extensor carpi ulnaris and the anconeus are then elevated off the remaining lateral elbow capsule and LCL complex with sharp dissection
- An effort should be made to preserve capsular flaps as the tendon graft is best left extra-articular by closing the capsular flaps underneath the graft at the end of the reconstruction
- The anterior capsule is opened laterally and the joint is entered

Bone tunnel preparation

- Next, the tunnels for insertion of the tendon graft into the ulna and humerus are created with a 4.0 mm high-speed burr
  - One hole of the ulnar tunnel is centered over the tubercle of the supinator crest, which can easily be palpated
  - The second hole is placed proximally and posteriorly, leaving a 1–1.5 cm bone bridge, wide enough to avoid a fracture
- A no. 2 suture is placed through the bone tunnel. It is grasped to select the isometric point on the surface of the humeral epicondyle, where the suture will maintain the same approximate tension during elbow flexion and extension
- The isometric point is located at the geometric center of the capitellar articular surface (**Figure 14.4**)

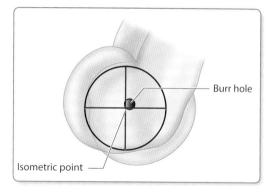

Figure 14.4 The isometric point is located at the geometric center of the capitellar articular surface on the surface of the humeral epicondyle.

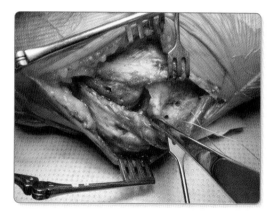

Figure 14.5 Sutures placed through the bone tunnels to be used as tendon graft passers.

- The first humeral tunnel is centered slightly proximal and posterior to the isometric point
- Next, two proximal exit holes are created on the anterior and posterior aspects of the lateral humeral column, converging toward the first humeral hole
- The anterior and posterior humeral tunnels are created
- Two no. 2 sutures are placed through these two tunnels, to be used as tendon graft passers (**Figure 14.5**)

Ligament reconstruction

Several options exist for tendon graft selection, including a palmaris longus autograft. Other autografts, e.g. plantaris or semitendinosus tendon, and triceps aponeurosis, can be used depending on the size of the patient.

- Two no. 2 FiberWires can be placed at the ends of the tendon graft in a running locking configuration to pull the tendon through the tunnels and assist in graft attachment
- The tendon graft is first passed through the ulnar tunnel with the no. 2 suture (**Figure 14.6**)
- The two ends of the tendon graft are first docked into the first humeral hole, and then into the anterior and posterior humeral tunnels using the two sutures (**Figure 14.7**)

- The sutures running into the tendon are then tied over the proximal aspect of the humeral epicondyle
- Usually, a no. 5 nonabsorbable suture is placed parallel to the tendon graft in the different bone tunnels to reinforce the construction (**Figure 14.8**)

Possible perioperative complications

- Care must be taken to avoid injuring the radial nerve distally around the supinator muscle and the radial neck
- The forearm must be positioned in pronation to increase the distance between the lateral surgical approach and the posterior interosseus nerve

Closure

- The remaining capsule should be sutured to seal the joint before the graft reconstruction is completed so that the graft remains extra-articular
- The graft should be tensioned with the joint in a reduced position, the forearm in full pronation, and the elbow in approximately 45° of flexion
- The tension may be increased by suturing the two limbs of the graft together at one or more points

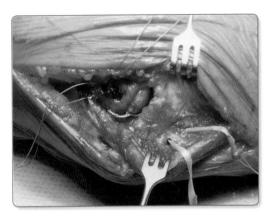

Figure 14.6 The tendon graft is passed through the ulnar tunnel.

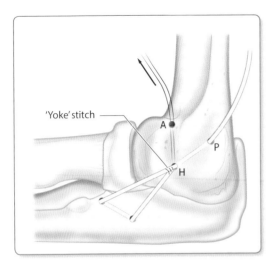

Figure 14.7 The two ends of the tendon graft are docked into the first humeral hole (H), and then into the anterior (A) and posterior (P) humeral tunnels.

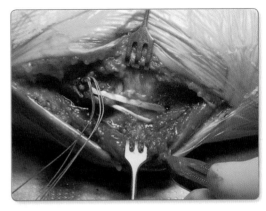

Figure 14.8 A nonabsorbable suture is placed parallel to the tendon graft in the different bone tunnels to reinforce the construction.

Postoperative management

- The ligamentous reconstruction needs to be protected for the first few weeks after surgery in order to prevent graft stretching and recurrent instability
- Initially after surgery, the elbow is immobilized in 90° of flexion and forearm pronation for 2 weeks
- Then motion is initiated with a hinge brace maintaining the forearm in pronation, and an extension block beyond 30°, for 4 weeks
- The hinge brace can then be maintained for a further 4 weeks, leaving the forearm free and removing the extension block
- Flexion–extension is performed with the forearm in pronation, and pronation–supination is performed with the elbow flexed to 90°
- Exercises to increase the strength of the extensor–supinator group also help stabilize the joint, and they may be initiated during the first few days after surgery
- Unrestricted activities are usually allowed 6 months after surgery

Outpatient follow-up

- Two weeks outpatient clinic review for wound inspection and change of splint
- Six weeks review for removal of splint and physiotherapy review
- Three-monthly review until patient has regained full range of movement, and resumed normal activities

Further reading

O'Driscoll SW, Spinner RJ, MacKee MD, et al. Tardy posterolateral rotatory instability of the elbow due to cubitus varus. J Bone Joint Surg Am 2001; 83:1358–1369.

Hall JA, McKee MD. Posterolateral rotatory instability of the elbow following radial head resection. J Bone Joint Surg Am 2005; 87:1571–1579.

Sanchez-Sotelo J, Morrey BF, O'Driscoll SW. Ligamentous repair and reconstruction for posterolateral rotatory instability of the elbow. J Bone Joint Surg Br 2005; 87:54–61.

Mansat P, Bonnevialle N. Luxations du coude. Appareil locomoteur 2009; 14-042-A-10.

Treatment of chronic medial elbow instability

Indications

- The symptoms of instability in athletes can occur following a single traumatic event or may be due to repetitive stress leading to chronic laxity, such as in a throwing athlete
- Patients with medial instability usually report medial elbow pain, decreased strength during overhead activity, and sometimes symptoms of ulnar neuropathy
- The athlete is most often exposed to severe, chronic repetitive valgus stresses. The anterior bundle is the most important stabilizer of the ulnar collateral ligament (UCL) complex for valgus throwing forces. The posterior oblique ligament functions with the elbow flexed beyond 90°
- Patients with isolated UCL injury often have pain slightly posterior to the common flexor origin, 2 cm distal to the medial epicondyle

Preoperative assessment

Clinical assessment

- Clinical examination should aim to assess the stability of the UCL complex, including the anterior oblique ligament, posterior oblique ligament, and transverse ligament (**Figure 15.1**)
- The most used and well-known test is the 'milking maneuver', which involves having the patient apply a valgus torque to the elbow by pulling down on the thumb of the injured extremity, with the contralateral limb providing stability:
  - With the modified milking maneuver, the examiner provides stability to the patient's elbow and pulls the thumb to create a valgus stress on the UCL. In cases of UCL insufficiency these tests result in pain and widening at the medial joint line

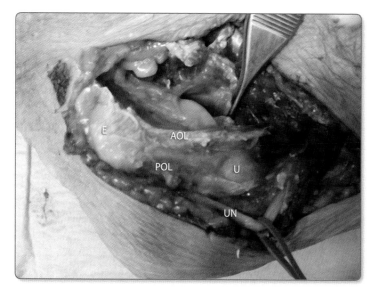

Figure 15.1 Medial collateral ligament and ulnar nerve. AOL, anterior oblique ligament; E, medial epicondyle; POL, posterior oblique ligament; U, ulna; UN, ulnar nerve.

- O'Driscoll and co-workers described the 'moving valgus stress test', in which the valgus torque is maintained constantly on the fully flexed elbow and then the elbow is rapidly extended:
  - This test is positive if medial elbow pain is elicited
  - The test has a 100% sensitivity and 75% specificity
- The abduction valgus stress test is performed by stabilizing the patient's abducted and externally rotated arm with the examiner's axilla and applying a valgus force to the elbow at 30° of flexion:
  - Testing with the forearm in neutral rotation has been shown to elicit the greatest valgus instability
  - A positive test results in medial elbow pain and widening along the medial joint line
  - Even so, valgus laxity can be subtle on physical examination, and the range of preoperative detection is between 26% and 82% of patients

Imaging assessment

- Anterior-posterior, lateral, and axillary views of the elbow are assessed for joint space narrowing, osteophytes, and loose bodies. Medial joint line opening can be measured utilizing valgus stress radiographs done manually or with commercially available devices. An opening of 3 mm has been considered diagnostic of valgus instability. Mild valgus elbow laxity, however, has been observed in uninjured, asymptomatic, dominant elbows of professional baseball pitchers
- CT and MRI can further diagnose loose bodies and osteophytes when suspected
- Conventional MRI can identify thickening within the ligament as a result of chronic injury or more obvious full thickness tears. MR arthrography enhanced with intra-articular gadolinium improves the diagnosis of partial undersurface tears
- Dynamic ultrasonography can detect increased laxity with valgus stress and has the advantage of being noninvasive, inexpensive, and dynamic

Timing for surgery

- UCL reconstruction is currently the best surgical choice for both acute and chronic UCL ruptures. Indications for reconstruction include:
  - Acute ruptures in high-level throwers
  - Significant chronic instability
  - Insufficient UCL tissue remaining after UCL debridement for calcifications, and
  - Recurrent pain and subtle valgus instability with throwing after supervised rehabilitation
- The probability of return to sports at the same pre-injury level following UCL rupture treated non-operatively is low (42% in one study) for overhead athletes. Therefore, for a high-level competitive thrower, surgical reconstruction is usually advocated

Surgical preparation

- The procedure is commonly performed under general anesthesia. An examination under anesthesia may be performed to confirm the diagnosis of medial instability of the elbow
- Preoperatively, the patient is assessed for presence of the palmaris longus tendon bilaterally. Of note, the palmaris longus tendon is unilaterally absent in 12–16%, and bilaterally absent in 9–27% of the general population. If absent, the gracilis, Achilles, plantaris, or fourth toe extensor tendon may be used. We prefer ipsilateral gracilis for ease of harvest

Surgical equipment

- Surgical equipment required for this procedure includes standard retractors and elevators for the elbow, drill bits and drill sleeves for the bone tunnels (typically 4.5 mm and 7.0 mm in diameter), and stout nonabsorbable suture material
- Optional equipment includes a tendon stripper for the free graft harvest, ligature passers to aid in threading the graft through the bone tunnels

Equipment positioning

- The surgeon stands at the right of the supine patient. An arm board is placed parallel to the operating table at the level of the arm
- All equipment is mounted a on portable rolling platform
- A mayo tray is on the left of the surgeon. An assistant stands to the left of surgeon

Patient positioning

- The patient is positioned supine on a well-padded table with a tourniquet placed on the upper arm, and the hand on a hand table or arm-board
- At the appropriate time, the autograft can be harvested. The ipsilateral leg should be prepared for harvesting of the gracilis. If the gracilis is required, it can be harvested with a tendon stripper after careful isolation of the graft from the other pes anserine tendons
- A tourniquet is applied to the proximal thigh but is not routinely used unless needed for harvesting
- A lateral post is used as a fulcrum to mantain the knee in the right position

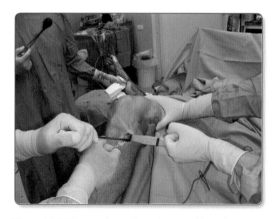

Figure 15.2 The gracilis tendon is harvested from the ipsilateral knee.

Surgical technique

Principles of surgical reconstruction

The different methods of UCL reconstruction proposed over the years by various authors have highlighted some surgical principles that are essential for anatomic and functional reconstruction:

- Minimize trauma to the flexor–pronator muscle group without transection from the medial epicondyle
- Reduce the incidence of ulnar nerve symptoms
- Use proximal and distal intraosseous fixation methods, i.e. tunnels
- Avoid interference of such tunnels or stitches with the course of the ulnar nerve
- Aim for anatomic reconstruction of both bands of the anterior oblique ligament (AOL)
- To have the possibility of fixing the two bands of the AOL independently with different tension at different degrees of flexion

Double-bundle technique using an autograft

- More recently, the authors presented a new double-bundle technique using gracilis from the ipsilateral knee (**Figure 15.2**), which simplifies graft passage, tensioning, and fixation
- The exposure is obtained by a muscle-splitting approach (**Figures 15.3** and **15.4**)
- The graft is prepared with a Krackow suture at the two ends of the tendon using a no. 2 Ti-Cron suture

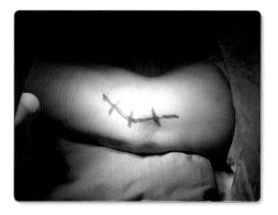

Figure 15.3 Planning the medial skin incision.

- A 7 mm drill hole is made at the sublime tubercle and directed toward the lateral and posterior cortex of the ulna, away from the proximal radioulnar joint (**Figure 15.5**). The far cortex is not breached
- The graft is folded over itself and introduced into the drill hole so at least 1 cm of the graft fills the drill hole (**Figure 15.6**)
- A 6–7 mm bioabsorbable interference screw is positioned in the drill hole to stabilize the graft (**Figure 15.7**)
- One 7 mm drill hole is positioned on the medial epicondyle at the most isometric point for the anterior bundle of the medial collateral ligament, i.e. at the anteroinferior surface of the medial epicondyle. This drill hole should not breach the far cortex and is oriented anterosuperiorly to avoid ulnar nerve damage

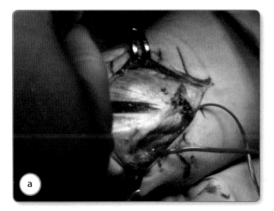

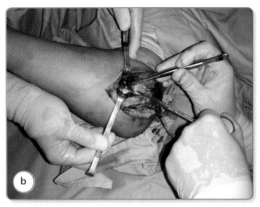

Figure 15.4 The exposure of the flexor pronator mass and muscle splitting approach (a,b) with ulnar nerve isolation (a).

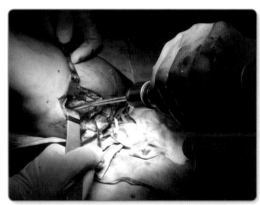

Figure 15.5 A 7 mm drill hole is placed in the sublime tubercle and directed toward the lateral and posterior cortex of the ulna, away from the proximal radioulnar joint.

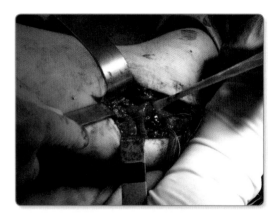

Figure 15.6 The graft is folded over itself and introduced into the drill hole so that at least 1 cm of the graft fills the drill hole.

- Two 4.5 mm drill holes are placed superiorly and independently convergent to the 7 mm graft hole away from the ulnar nerve
- The two ends of the tendon first pass together into the 7 mm graft hole. Then each single bundle is retrieved through the 4–5 mm drill hole (**Figure 15.8**) and sutured over itself at different degrees of flexion: anterior bundle at 30° and posterior bundle at 70° (**Figure 15.9**)
- After the tendon has been sutured, the fascia is used to cover the new tissue (**Figure 15.10**)
- This technique allows the reconstruction of a new ligament tenseiond in the arc of motion and thick enough to reproduce the original UCL

Possible perioperative complications

- The most common complications are ulnar or medial antebrachial nerve dysfunction (often transient), stiffness, medial epicondyle fracture, and nonspecific elbow pain

Postoperative management

- Postoperatively, the elbow is placed in a brace for 6 weeks, and rehabilitative protocols start at 2 weeks
- Sporting activities are initiated at 3–4 months, and a return to pre-injury sporting levels is allowed at 6–8 months postoperatively

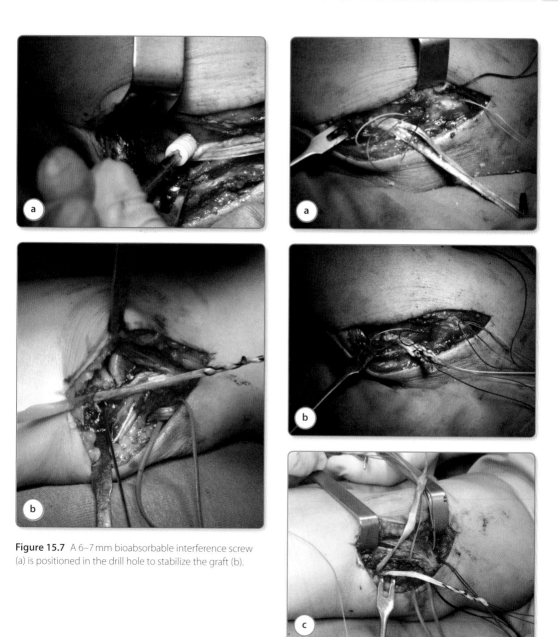

Figure 15.7 A 6–7 mm bioabsorbable interference screw (a) is positioned in the drill hole to stabilize the graft (b).

Figure 15.8 Two 4.5 mm drill holes are placed superiorly and independently convergent to the 7 mm graft hole away from the ulnar nerve (a). The two ends of the tendon first pass together into the 7 mm graft hole (b), and then each single bundle is retrieved through the 4–5 mm drill hole (c).

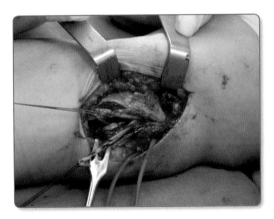

Figure 15.9 The two ends of the tendon are sutured over themselves at different degrees of flexion: anterior bundle at 30° and posterior bundle at 70°.

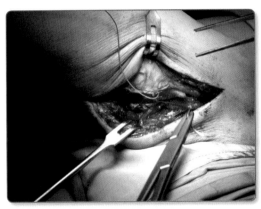

Figure 15.10 After suturing the tendon, the fascia is used to cover the new tissue.

Further reading

Ahmad CS, ElAttrache NS. Elbow valgus instability in the throwing athlete. J Am Acad Orthop Surg 2006; 14:693–700.

Altchek DW, Andrew JR. Medial collateral ligament injuries. In: Altchek DW, Andrew JR (eds), The athlete's elbow. Philadelphia: Lippincott Williams & Wilkins, 2001:153–173.

Murthi AM, Keener JD, Armstrong AD, Getz CL. The recurrent unstable elbow: diagnosis and treatment. Instr Course Lect 2011; 60:215–226.

O'Driscoll SWM, Lawton RL, Smith AM. The moving valgus stress test for medial collateral ligament tears of the elbow. Am J Sports Med 2005; 33:231–239.

Open debridement for elbow arthritis

Indications

- Elbow arthritis is a debilitating condition in which a painful and stiff joint is more common than it is in other arthropathies
- Primary osteoarthritis is rare while trauma and rheumatoid arthritis are the causes in the vast majority of cases
- Activities of daily living can be sufficiently accomplished with an arc of motion of 100° (from 30° of extension to 130° of flexion), and 100° for rotation (50° of pronation to 50° of supination)
- Surgery is indicated in patients < 60 years old with moderate pain at the end points of motion

Preoperative assessment

Patient history

- Mechanical impingement-type pain at terminal flexion–extension with some degree of terminal extension loss in the early stages of the disease
- Pain in the mid-arc motion and a greater degree of motion loss in the late stages of the disease
- Occasionally nerve deficit from ulnar entrapment neuropathy
- Related to level of activity and occupation:
  - Primary arthritis is commonly seen in throwing athletes, weight lifters, and middle-aged manual laborers who subject their elbows to high force loads
- Known history of rheumatoid arthritis, hemophilia, osteochondritis dissecans, ligamentous insufficiency, or crystalline arthropathy
- Post-traumatic arthritis:
  - Detailed information regarding previous surgery, position of any hardware, and history of infection

Physical examination

- Skin inspection for any surgical incisions, scars, or areas of fibrosis
- Active and passive range of motion of the elbow and forearm, measured carefully with a goniometer bilaterally
- Crepitus
- 'Catching' or 'locking' from loose bodies
- Varus, valgus, or rotational instability, assessed to determine collateral ligament insufficiency
- Evaluation of ulnar nerve function
- Aspiration of synovial fluid when there is a suspicion of infection; complete blood cell count, erythrocyte sedimentation rate, and C-reactive protein level are needed

Imaging assessment

Radiographs

- Anteroposterior, lateral with the elbow flexed to 90°, and radiocapitellar oblique views are taken:
  - Radiographic findings in rheumatoid arthritis include symmetric joint space narrowing, bone resorption, and disuse osteopenia without osteophyte formation
  - The unique findings in elbow arthritis are preservation of the articular cartilage and maintenance of the radiocapitellar and ulnohumeral joint spaces even in the advanced stages of primary arthritis
  - Osteophytes and loose bodies at the olecranon and coronoid process, extending into the fossae, are typically seen

Radiographic classification of primary elbow osteoarthritis

- Class I: marginal arthritic spurring of the ulnotrochlear joint with a normal radiocapitellar joint
- Class II: ulnotrochlear degenerative changes plus arthritic changes in the radiocapitellar joint without subluxation

- Class III: the arthritic changes of class I and II with the simultaneous presence of radial head subluxation

Computed tomography (CT) with three-dimensional reconstruction

- Useful in cases of heterotopic ossification
- Helpful in identifying hidden osteophytes in the fossae, in the posterior capitellum, and adjacent to the ulnar nerve in the medial gutter

Other investigations

- Electro diagnostic studies for ulnar nerve dysfunction or cervical radiculopathy affecting the elbow region
- Bone scans, MRI, and cultures in case of infection and septic arthritis

Surgical preparation

Surgical equipment

- Hohmann retractors and Cobb elevators
- Osteotomes (straight, curved), burrs, curretes, and rongeurs
- Drill, neurosurgical dowel or trephine, and saw

Patient positioning

- General or regional anesthesia is used
- Intravenous antibiotic prophylaxis is given prior to the skin incision in line with local hospital policy and guidelines
- The limb is prepared and draped to the axilla with a tourniquet applied as proximally as possible, which is inflated to 250 mmHg
- The patient is positioned on the operating table according to the surgeon's preference and the surgical approach being used

Surgical technique

Operative treatment with open debridement

Basic steps

- Patients with pain throughout the entire range of motion and diffuse joint space narrowing are more likely to benefit from interpositional arthroplasty or total elbow arthroplasty
- Open debridement seems to be superior to arthroscopic debridement in cases of heterotopic ossification, great deformity, or a

previously operated elbow, as in cases of ulnar nerve transposition
- Ulnar nerve decompression is indicated in the presence of ulnar neuritis and in patients with limited elbow extension (>60°) and flexion (≤100°)
- Extension is restored by:
  - Removal of loose bodies from the olecranon fossa
  - Resection of osteophytes from the tip of the olecranon
  - Release of the anterior capsule
- Flexion is restored by:
  - Release of the posterior capsule
  - Resection of the anterior bony impingement between the coronoid and coronoid fossa, and the radial head and radial fossa

Surgical approaches

- Open synovectomy with or without radial head excision in rheumatoid arthritis
- Ulnohumeral arthroplasty (Outerbridge–Kashiwagi procedure)
- Lateral column approach
- Medial approach

Ulnohumeral arthroplasty (Figure 16.1)

Indications

- There are limited indications in cases of primary and post-traumatic arthritis due to mechanical impingement from osteophyte formation at the coronoid process or olecranon
- It is not indicated for rheumatoid arthritis
- There is limited access to the radiocapitellar space

Technique

- The patient is positioned in a lateral decubitus or prone position with all bony prominences well padded. The upper arm is supported by a padded post so that the elbow can be freely flexed beyond 90°
- Make a posterior longitudinal incision that is slightly curved round the olecranon tip and starts 6–8 cm proximally to and extend to 4 cm distal to the tip
- The triceps fascia is identified and the triceps tendon is incised longitudinally in its midline. The posterior aspect of the elbow in then

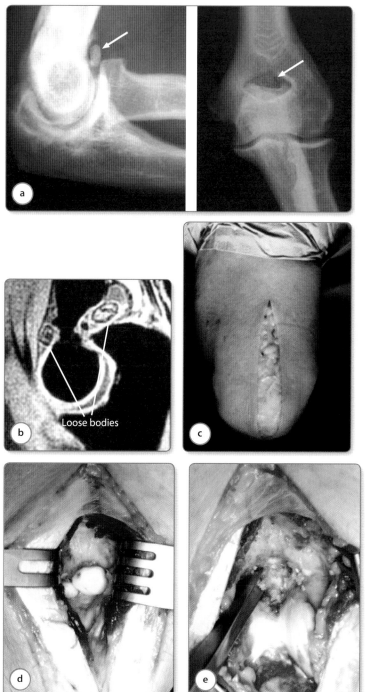

Figure 16.1 A 67-year-old man with elbow stiffness and a loose body treated with the Outerbridge–Kashiwagi procedure. (a) Preoperative radiographs showing loose bodies (arrowed) in the olecranon and coronoid fossae. (b) CT confirming the radiographic diagnosis. (c) Midline posterior incision revealing the fascia over the triceps tendon. (d) The olecranon fossa with the loose body is identified through the fibers of the triceps muscle. (e) The loose body is removed and the olecranon fossa is debrided. (f) The olecranon fossa is trephined and the loose body in the coronoid fossa is identified. (g) The loose body is removed and the coronoid fossa is debrided.

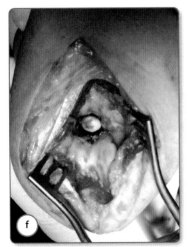
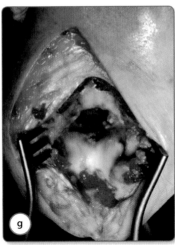

Figure 16.1 *Continued*

visualized. Alternatively, the triceps can be reflected medially, an approach that is particularly useful when the ulnar nerve needs to be decompressed
- Capsulotomy is performed and posterior osteophytes are removed using an osteotome or an oscillating saw. A rongeur is used to smooth the edges
- A 1.5 cm neurosurgical dowel or trephine is centered on the olecranon fossa aiming anteriorly and cephalad by 15–20°, following the curvature of the trochlea
- Fenestrate the olecranon fossa until the anterior cortex is perforated. Widen the hole using curettes to ensure adequate visualization of the coronoid process when the elbow is maximally flexed
- Remove all osteophytes from the coronoid process using an osteotome introduced through the humeral window. Anterior loose bodies can be visualized and removed
- The anterior capsule can be stripped from the anterior humerus using a blunt periosteal elevator to gain better elbow extension
- Manipulate the elbow to maximize the total range of motion
- Bone wax can be used to cover the margins of the foramen, and Gelfoam to occupy the dead space
- The wound is copiously irrigated and closed in standard fashion. A drain is used to avoid postoperative hematomas, and is removed on the 2nd postoperative day

Lateral column approach (Figure 16.2)

Indications
- This approach is preferred for radiocapitellar joint and fossa pathology
- It is used when there is no indication for ulnar nerve transposition

Technique
- The patient is positioned supine with the arm placed on an arm board
- A limited Kocher's incision is performed starting from the supracondylar ridge of the humerus and progressing distally across the lateral epicondyle towards the radial head
- Brachialis is elevated from the supracondylar ridge proximally, and the interval between extensor carpi radialis longus and brevis is developed distally
- The anterior capsule is visualized and excised, while the lateral collateral ligament is protected under the remainder of the common extensor
- The coronoid and radial fossa are debrided and coronoid process osteophyte and loose bodies are removed
- Be careful not to destabilize the elbow with overzealous coronoid process debridement
- Radial head excision should be considered in cases of restricted forearm rotation, tenderness over the radial head, or radiographic evidence of radiocapitellar arthritis (**Figure 16.3**).

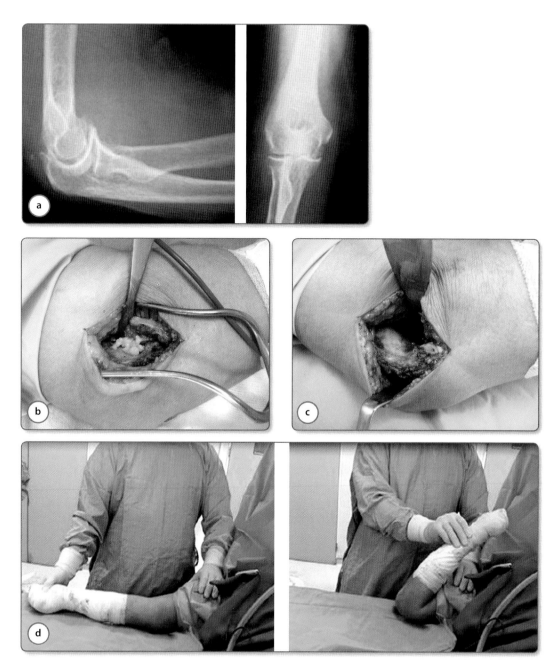

Figure 16.2 A 60-year-old woman with elbow stiffness. (a) Preoperative radiographs showing osteophytes at the olecranon tip and coronoid process. (b) After a limited Kocher exposure, loose bodies are removed from the anterior compartment. (c) Using the same skin incision, the posterior capsule is excised and the posterior compartment is debrided. (d) The elbow is manipulated through the full range of motion to check if any mechanical impingement is still present.

Pronate the forearm to avoid iatrogenic injury to the posterior interosseous nerve, and excise the radial head to improve the functional outcome

- Posterior capsule inspection and release can be accomplished via the same skin incision or alternatively via a second minimal posterior longitudinal incision
- The deep fascia between anconeus and extensor carpi ulnaris is incised
- The anconeus and triceps are reflected posteriorly from the supracondylar ridge with a Hohmann retractor, taking care not damage the lateral collateral ligament
- The posterior ulnohumeral joint is now exposed
- Any synovitis and capsular contracture can be excised
- Any impinging osteophytes can be removed from the tip of the olecranon and olecranon fossa using a narrow osteotome or a rongeur

- It is important not to be overzealous with posterior bone resection in the presence of lack of full extension. Contracture of the anterior capsule is likely to be the cause
- After thorough irrigation, the wounds are closed in a layered fashion

Medial approach

Indications

- This is preferred in cases of ulnar neuropathy when ulnar decompression or transposition is required
- It is also used in cases of ulnohumeral pathology when the radiocapitellar joint does not need to be addressed

Technique

- The patient is placed supine with the arm positioned on an arm board
- A medial, slightly curvilinear incision is made, centered on the medial epicondyle

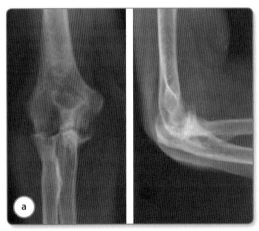

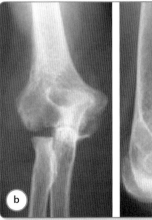
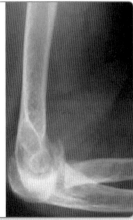

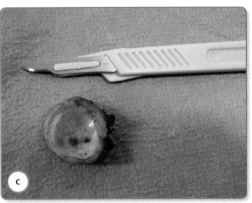

Figure 16.3 A 55-year-old woman with rheumatoid arthritis of the elbow. (a) Preoperative radiographs showing advanced radiocapitellar arthritis. (b) Radial head excision was performed. (c) Postoperative radiographs.

- Care is taken to preserve the terminal branches of the medial cutaneous nerve of the forearm
- The ulnar nerve is dissected free from the arcade of Struthers and the fascia of flexor carpi ulnaris, and mobilized anteriorly
- The triceps is elevated from the intermuscular septum and humerus
- The posterior oblique bundle of the medial collateral ligament is identified and excised, and the medial side of the elbow joint is exposed
- The posteromedial capsule is excised and any osteophytes in the ulnohumeral joint or medial gutter are removed
- Osteophytes beneath the anterior bundle of the medial collateral ligament are removed with the elbow flexed
- The fascia of the pronator flexor muscle group is incised at its center
- The brachialis muscle is dissected off the humerus proximally
- Distally, the flexor pronator mass is divided parallel to its fibers with a 1.5 cm span of flexor carpi ulnaris tendon left attached to the medial epicondyle (Hotchkiss's 'over-the-top' approach). Alternatively, an interneural plane can be created between the flexor carpi ulnaris and palmaris longus (the medial trans flexor approach)
- The brachialis muscle and pronator flexor muscle group are elevated anteriorly as a single soft tissue sleeve
- The anterior bundle of the medial collateral ligament lying under the humeral head of flexor carpi ulnaris is by the surgeon protected while the anterior capsule is incised
- With the elbow flexed any coronoid osteophytes are excised, and with the elbow in extension the coronoid fossa is deepened using an osteotome and a burr
- The elbow is taken through a full range of motion, and any persisting impingement is identified and managed
- Anterior subcutaneous transposition of the ulnar nerve is performed and the wound closed in standard fashion

- An additional lateral approach is indicated in the following circumstances:
  - A radial fossa that is not well visualized using the medial transflexor approach
  - Lateral pain preoperatively
  - Loose bodies in the posterior radiocapitellar compartment
  - When procedures on the medial side of the elbow are inadequate to increase the range of motion

Possible perioperative complications

- Late supracondylar fractures with improper placement of the humeral foraminectomy
- Recurrence, with a rate of < 10%
- Postoperative ulnar neuropathy
- Postoperative hematomas with large soft tissue flaps when drains are not used
- Median and radial nerve palsy

Postoperative management

- Apply a long arm posterior splint with the forearm in neutral and the elbow in 20° of extension for 1 week
- An active range of motion is allowed one 1 week after the splint has been removed
- Prophylaxis for heterotopic ossification includes oral indomethacin (indometacin) 25 mg three times daily for 2 weeks

Results

- There is 75–80% success at mid-term follow-up, with restoration of motion and alleviation of pain
- The improvement in the range of motion is expected to be around 20–30°
- Longer-term outcome studies have shown a measurable loss of range of motion and recurrence of osteophytes over time

Further reading

Cheung EV, Adams R, Morrey BF. Primary osteoarthritis of the elbow: current treatment options. J Am Acad Orthop Surg 2008; 16:77–87.

Gallo RA, Payatakes A, Sotereanos DG. Surgical options for the arthritic elbow. J Hand Surg Am 2008; 33:746–759.

Papatheodorou LK, Baratz ME, Sotereanos DG. Elbow arthritis: current concepts. J Hand Surg Am 2013; 38:605–613.

17 Arthroscopic arthrolysis of the elbow

Indications

- Most daily activities can be performed with a flexion and extension arc of 100°, and rotation of 100° at the elbow. More severe restriction is mostly associated with a considerable loss of function
- Post-traumatic conditions are the main cause of elbow stiffness. Other causes of stiffness are primary arthritis, rheumatoid arthritis, septic arthritis, osteochondritis, and secondary arthritis
- The main indication for release of the elbow is a painful and stiff elbow. It should, however, be realized that moderately stiff elbows can be very painful and very stiff elbows can be pain free
- The use of an arthroscope in releases is limited to intra-articular causes of stiffness including:
  - Capsular contractures
  - Synovial swelling
  - Arthritic lesions and osteophytes
  - Loose bodies
  - Intra-articular adhesions
- Relative contra indications to arthrocopic release are:
  - Previous elbow procedures with altered anatomy, e.g. ulnar nerve transposition
  - Post-traumatic conditions with incongruent articular surfaces, where motion will not be restored even after a release
  - Septic conditions
  - Extra-articular conditions including heterotopic bone formation and skin contractures

Preoperative assessment

Clinical assessment

- The patient describes stiffness with or without pain. Locking symptoms suggest a loose body (**Figure 17.1**)
- During examination, the range of motion is compared with the contralateral side

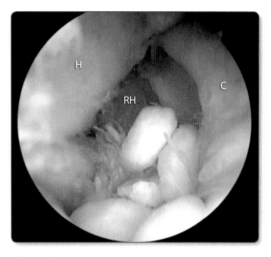

Figure 17.1 Loose bodies in the ventral compartment. C, capsule; H, humerus; RH, radial head.

- Use of a goniometer is advised to enable an accurate comparison with the postoperative final assessment
- The rotations of the forearm should also be measured

Imaging assessment

- Anteroposterior and lateral radiographs are generally sufficient to establish the pathology. Further oblique projections can be helpful
- CT with three-dimensional reconstruction, as well as MRI, is helpful to visualize the extent of osteophytes, heterotopic ossifications, and the location of loose bodies (**Figure 17.2**)
- CT is also useful in imaging post fracture deformities

Timing for surgery

- The timing for surgery is based on persistent symptoms of incapacitating stiffness with or without pain as well as locking or pseudo-locking

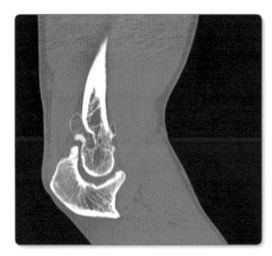

Figure 17.2 CT of an arthritic elbow with osteophytes on the ventral humerus as well as the olecranon tip. The dorsal aspect of the olecranon fossa is completely covered by an osteophyte.

Surgical preparation

Surgical equipment

- A standard arthroscopic setup consists of a camera system, a pump, and a shaver. The procedure is normally performed with standard arthroscopic equipment
- The pump pressure should be kept as low as possible. A release of the elbow is a time-consuming procedure, and long-term high pressures can cause significant swelling in the surrounding tissues that may limit the surgery
- Both a small (2.7 mm) as well as a large (4.5 mm) diameter arthroscope are helpful
- Two types of shaver blades are needed: incisor blades for resection of soft tissue and a burr for removal of osteophytes. Some blades, e.g. the 'bone cutter' blade of Smith and Nephew, combine both functions
- A radiofrequency device is useful if used with care to avoid neurovascular damage
- Small retractors can be helpful in the ventral compartment to retract the ventral capsule and brachial muscle
- Arthroscopic punches or scissors are useful in cutting thickened capsule. It is important to leave one part of the scissors or punch inside the joint to prevent cutting adjacent tissues
- Periosteal elevators are helpful in detaching capsule from the bone

- In cases of previous ulnar nerve transposition, it is mandatory to locate the new course of the nerve either by a small exploration or by ultrasonography

Equipment positioning

- While the patient is mostly positioned in lateral decubitus or prone position, the arthroscopic tower is placed at the other side of the table
- The instruments, and the nurse, are positioned next to the surgeon; the instruments can also be put on a small instrument table, placed over the patient

Patient positioning

- After inducing general anesthesia, preferably in combination with an interscalene block, the patient is positioned in a lateral decubitus, prone, or supine position
- A tourniquet is used to enable better vision in the joint during surgery. The pressure should not exceed 100 mmHg more than the systolic blood pressure. The upper arm with the tourniquet is positioned on an arm holder (**Figure 17.3**). In this position the elbow is

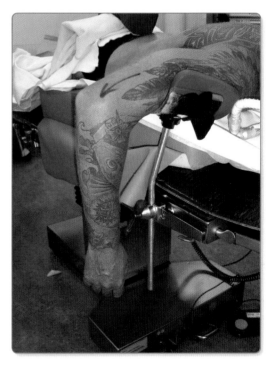

Figure 17.3 Patient in the prone position with the right arm on a support.

freely movable. It is important to check if the elbow in this position can be flexed as much as possible during surgery, creating a wider exposure in the joint as well as the possibility to test the achieved excursion after the release

- Some surgeons prefer the supine position, with traction on the hand and the elbow hanging free in 90° of flexion. The disadvantage of this position is that the elbow is not as movable as in the previous position without taking the arm out of the traction
- During positioning, care should be taken to prevent pressure on nerves, e.g. the peroneal nerve and ulnar nerve
- Pressure on the lateral cutaneous nerve of the thigh should be avoided in the lateral decubitus position. In the prone position, the chest and abdomen should be free, which can be achieved with cylindrical pillows under the shoulders and pelvis. Extreme abduction of the arm should be avoided to prevent stretching of the brachial plexus

Further preparation

- It is important to maintain orientation, especially in the prone patient
- It is advisable to mark the course of the ulnar nerve and the portals to be used

- Antibiotics are advised for this frequently time-consuming procedure
- It is advised to administer indomethacin (indometacin) or other nonsteroidal anti-inflammatory drugs to prevent heterotopic ossification

Surgical technique
Portals and inspection of the joint

- Normal saline is injected through the distal posterolateral portal in the 'soft area' (**Figure 17.4**). The elbow extends when enough pressure has been achieved inside the joint. When the joint is very stiff, an alternative route to instil fluid is the antero lateral portal, about 1 cm ventral and distal to the lateral epicondyle, aiming obliquely in relation to the joint
- The safest entry for the arthroscope is through the proximal medial portal, ventrally from the intermuscular septum (**Figure 17.5**). After a small skin incision has been made, the septum can be palpated with the blunt trocar, and, directing the trocar ventrally to the septum following the ventral aspect of the humerus, the distended capsule can be perforated
- If the joint is too stiff to allow entry medially, the anterolateral portal can be used to

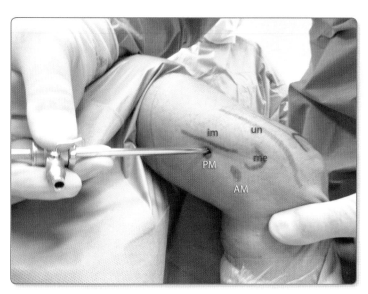

Figure 17.4　The trocar is inserted through the proximal medial portal, ventral to the intermuscular septum. AM, anteromedial portal; im, intermuscular septum; me, medial epicondyle; PM, proximal medial portal; un, ulnar nerve.

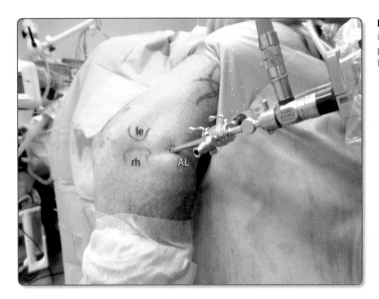

Figure 17.5 The arthroscope is introduced through the anterolateral portal. AL, anterolateral portal; le, lateral epicondyle; rh, radial head.

introduce the scope. A thorough inspection of the ventral joint area can be performed

- If it is not possible to enter the joint and the scope remains outside the joint, indicated by the presence of the white capsule at one side and the red brachialis muscle on the other side, the shaver can be inserted from the distal medial portal
- As long as the shaver tip can be seen from are just outside the joint, it is possible to resect the capsule from outside. This should always be done under vision. Blind shaving involves a risk of damaging neurovascular structures
- In stiff elbows it is generally better to accomplish the surgery in the ventral compartment before continuing the inspection posteriorly
- The next step is to insert the scope posterolaterally through the soft spot. In stiff elbows the smaller scope is preferred. Just adacent to this portal, 3–5 mm laterally, a second portal can be used to insert a shaver or other instruments (**Figure 17.5**)
- Alternatively, when using a large arthroscope, a more distal ulnar portal can be used for the scope and the soft spot portal for the surgery
- Through this portal, the dorsal capitellum can be inspected, as can the dorsal proximal radioulnar joint and the ulnohumeral joint
- The proximal posterior compartment around the olecranon fossa can be approached by making a trans-tricipital portal. The fossa is

palpated with a needle. A small longitudinal incision is made through the triceps tendon over the center of the fossa

- The adhesions can be disrupted with the blunt trocar, following which the arthroscope is inserted. An alternative route is the proximal posterolateral portal, 2–3 cm lateral to the previous portal, and just lateral to the triceps tendon (**Figure 17.5**). Both portals are necessary to perform surgery in the posterior compartment

Procedure

- It is generally advisable to start surgery in the ventral compartment; swelling of the soft tissue after lengthy surgical procedures is more serious ventrally than dorsally, and makes surgery more difficult
- If it is possible to visualize the joint surface, the surgeon should start to remove blocking osteophytes in osteoarthritis
- If it is impossible to enter the joint, the surgeon should start with a capsulotomy as described above
- When osteophytes have to be removed, surgery should start on the coronoid process (**Figure 17.6**). A burr or a small 5 mm osteotome can be used. Sometimes these osteophytes extend into the proximal radioulnar joint and block forearm rotation. They should be removed if they impair rotation (**Figure 17.11**)

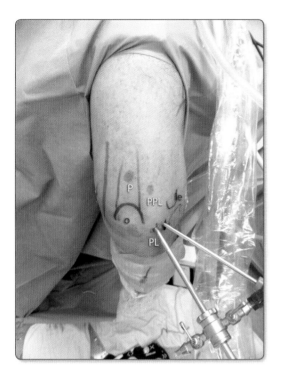

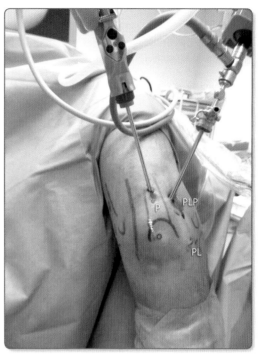

Figure 17.6 The arthroscope and shaver are inserted through both posterolateral portals. le, lateral epicondyle; o, olecranon; P, posterior portal through the triceps tendon; PL, two posterolateral portals through the soft spot; PPL, proximal posterolateral portal, adjacent to the triceps tendon.

Figure 17.7 The arthroscope is introduced through the proximal posterolateral portal, and the shaver through the posterior portal. o, olecranon; P, posterior portal; PL, posterolateral portals through the soft spot; PLP, proximal posterolateral portal.

- Osteophytes on the ventral distal humeral surface should also be removed if they block full flexion
- The next step is to perform a capsulotomy or capsulectomy
- It is easiest to start to detach the capsule from the humerus, with either a shaver or a small elevator (**Figure 17.7**). The aim is to achieve full extension
- Under direct vision from the medial side, the capsule is split from lateral to medial (**Figure 17.8**). As the deep branch of the radial nerve is close to the capsule, it is advisable to start dividing the capsule laterally
- A shaver with low suction is used. The opening of the blade should always be directed obliquely along the capsule and remain under vision, and never be directed toward the muscle. A rather extensive capsulectomy can be achieved

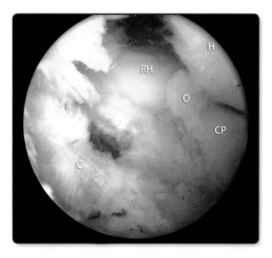

Figure 17.8 Osteophyte between the radial head and coronoid process. C, capsule; CP, coronoid process; H, humerus; O, osteophyte; RH, radial head.

- If full extension cannot be achieved, either the capsulectomy was insufficient, or structures including osteophytes and scar tissue in the olecranon fossa are preventing full extension
- After the ventral compartment, continue with the releases in the posterolateral corner. Both adjacent portals in the soft spot can be used. All scar tissue in this area can be removed through these portals, as well as osteophytes blocking rotations in the dorsal part of the proximal radioulnar joint
- The next step is to address the proximal posterior compartment. Scoping through the trans-tricipital portal, the shaver can be introduced through the proximal posterolateral portal (**Figure 17.9**). The capsule can be detached from the dorsal humerus with the shaver, bearing in mind the position of the ulnar nerve. A periosteal elevator is safer for the ulnar nerve when staying on bone. A complete capsulectomy is generally not needed in this compartment. Large osteophytes in the olecranon fossa as well as around the tip of the olecranon prevent full extension and should be removed (**Figure 17.10**)
- Osteophytes in the medial recess are close to the ulnar nerve and should be carefully approached. Both the medial and lateral recesses are inspected for loose bodies

- Adhesions preventing motion should be addressed
- After completing the decompression, the range of motion should be recorded, although swelling of the joint might limit the range of motion
- During surgery with a tourniquet, bleeding is not a serious problem
- A radiofrequency device can be used, respecting the proximity of the neurovascular structures
- As the joint is close to the skin, portals should be closed and a standard pressure bandage applied

Possible perioperative complications

- Generally, these are related to the anesthesia or positioning
- Local complications include:
  - Vascular: The brachial artery is potentially in danger, although as it runs ventral to the brachial muscle, the muscle protects the artery
  - Neurologic: Two nerves run close to the joint:
    - Dorsally, the ulnar nerve runs just outside the ulnar gutter. Medial portal placement should be accurate to avoid the nerve.

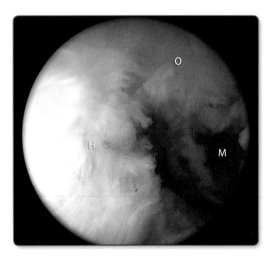

Figure 17.9 Lateral view of patient in Figure 17.2 with the humerus with overhanging osteophyte, capsule partly removed, and visible brachialis muscle. H, humerus; M, muscle; O, osteophyte.

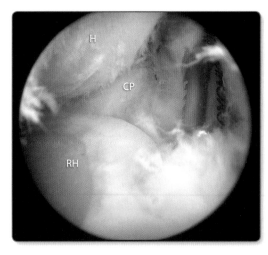

Figure 17.10 Lateral view with the shaver directed toward the capsule and away from the muscle. CP, coronoid process; H, humerus; RH, radial head.

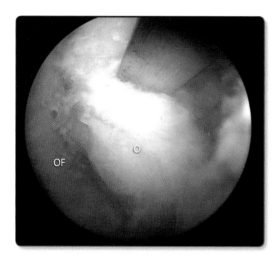

Figure 17.11 Olecranon fossa view of the same patient as shown in Figure 17.2 with osteophytes removed by an osteotome. O, osteophyte; OF, olecranon fossa.

Drawing the course of the nerve will help in protecting the nerve

- The deep branch of the radial nerve (mainly motor) runs ventrally, close to the capsule, at the level of the radial head. The superficial branch (mainly sensory) runs more ventrally and should be avoided when making the anterolateral portal. Injury can be avoided by opening the subcutaneous layer and capsule with a small clamp before inserting the scope, taking care to direct the scope obliquely toward the joint line and not parallel to it

Closure

- The joint is in close proximity to the skin. For this reason it is better to close the portals to prevent drainage, potentially leading to infection. A standard pressure bandage is applied

Postoperative management

- The arm is put in a sling for 1 week, and daily passive exercises should start immediately postoperatively under physiotherapy guidance
- If extension loss was the main problem, the elbow should be immobilized in a removable splint that can be removed for daily exercises
- Adequate pain relief should be provided

Outpatient follow-up

- Frequent follow-up is needed to monitor early recurrence of stiffness that can be treated by increasing physiotherapy or manipulation under anesthesia
- In releasing stiffness from soft tissue contractures, a near-normal function can be expected. In osteoarthritic osteophyte removal, the function can be improved but will never return to normal

Further reading

Ball CM, Meunier M, Galatz LM, Yamaguchi K. Arthroscopic treatment of post-traumatic elbow contracture. J Shoulder Elbow Surg 2002; 11:624–629.

Stanley D, Trail I (eds). Operative Elbow Surgery. Edinburgh: Churchill Livingstone, 2012.

Total elbow arthroplasty without bone loss

Indications

- The indications for an unlinked total elbow arthroplasty are similar to those for any design of elbow arthroplasty. The necessary prerequisites for an unlinked implant are:
    - The presence of sufficient bone stock to support the implant. In the absence of sufficient bone stock or ligamentous constraints, a linked arthroplasty should be used
    - Intact medial and lateral collateral ligaments
    - The presence of functioning and balanced elbow flexor and extensor muscles to maintain implant stability
- Typical indications include inflammatory arthritis (rheumatoid, psoriatic, hemophilic), primary or post-traumatic osteoarthritis, osteonecrosis, periarticular tumors, and comminuted distal humeral articular fractures in elderly patients
- Active infection is an absolute contraindication to elbow arthroplasty. The absence of functioning muscles to move the elbow and a nonfunctional hand are relative contraindications. Patients who are unwilling to live within the activity and weight restrictions, which are thought to be needed for implant longevity, should be managed with an alternative treatment
- Poor skin quality must be corrected before or at the same time as the arthroplasty

Preoperative assessment

Clinical assessment

- Skin quality, previous incisions, range of motion, and neurovascular status must be evaluated
- Any sign of infection must be noted
- The wrist and the shoulder must also be assessed

Imaging assessment

- Usually, plain anteroposterior and lateral radiographs of the elbow are sufficient prior to a total elbow arthroplasty
- The joint line, deformity, and bone stock must be analyzed
- Previous hardware or previous prosthesis can be also noted

Surgical preparation

Surgical equipment

- Ancillary prosthesis
- Implants of all available sizes
- Bone saw
- High-speed 2 mm and 5 mm burr
- Low viscosity cement with antibiotics
- Special gun and nozzle for cement injection
- Cement restrictors (for humerus and ulna)
- Suture-passer

Equipment positioning

- Instruments table should be positioned on the operating side
- Surgeon and nurse stand on the operating elbow side
- Assistant on the opposite side of the table stabilizes the forearm of the operating elbow

Patient positioning

- The patient is positioned supine with a sandbag under the scapula, and the arm is draped free with a non sterile tourniquet and brought across the chest
- Some surgeons preferred the lateral decubitus position (**Figure 18.1**)

Timing for surgery

- Surgery is planned following a careful evaluation of the patient
- Any sites of infection must be ruled out

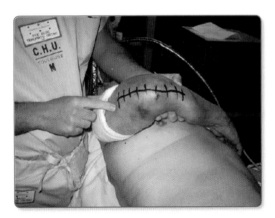

Figure 18.1 The patient can be placed in the lateral decubitus position.

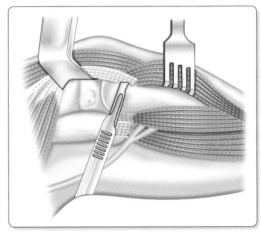

Figure 18.2 The triceps is elevated subperiosteally from its attachment on the ulna in the triceps-reflecting approach.

Surgical technique

Exposure

- A posterior longitudinal midline incision is made just lateral to the tip of the olecranon
- Full-thickness flaps are elevated. The extent of flap elevation is based on how the triceps is to be managed surgically
- The ulnar nerve is identified, protected with help of a Penrose drain, and transposed anteriorly

Triceps management

- The surgical management of the triceps is a matter of surgeon preference, and includes triceps-sparing, triceps-reflecting, and triceps-splitting approaches
  - *Triceps-reflecting approach:* The triceps is elevated subperiosteally from its attachment on the ulna from medial to lateral; it must be carefully protected and reattached post operatively. Surgical exposure is facilitated with this approach (**Figure 18.2**)
  - *Triceps-splitting approach:* A midline split is made in the triceps muscle and tendon that is carried distally onto the subcutaneous border of the ulna between the anconeus and the flexor carpi ulnaris (**Figure 18.3**). The medial triceps is elevated in continuity with the flexor carpi ulnaris, while the

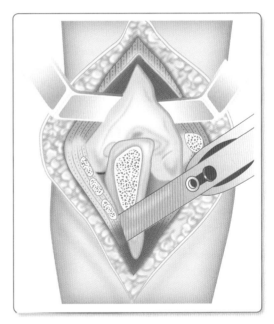

Figure 18.3 A triceps-splitting approach with a midline split in the triceps muscle and tendon that is carried distally onto the subcutaneous border of the ulna.

lateral triceps is elevated in continuity with the anconeus. The medial collateral ligament and lateral collateral ligament complex are tagged and released from their humeral attachments. The shoulder is externally rotated and the elbow is flexed, allowing the ulna to separate from the humerus

– *Triceps-sparing approach:* The triceps is left attached to the tip of the olecranon. This approach was initially described for total elbow arthroplasty in the context of distal humeral fracture, but it can be used for other indications. This approach prevents triceps weakness post operatively, but the surgical exposure is limited (**Figure 18.4**)

Surgical technique for the linked Coonrad–Morrey prosthesis (Zimmer)

Humerus preparation

- The mid-portion of the trochlea is removed with an oscillating saw up to the roof of the olecranon fossa
- The roof of the olecranon is entered with a burr, and a small twist reamer is used to identify the humeral medullary canal
- An alignment stem is then placed down the canal and the humeral cutting guide is positioned
- An oscillating saw is used to make cuts along the edges of the jig, with the tip of the saw pointing away from the midline of the humerus to avoid crosshatching at the junction of the column and the olecranon fossa
- Progressive 10 cm rasps are then used to calibrate the canal
- The anterior capsule is completely subperiosteally released from the anterior aspect of the humerus to accommodate the anterior flange of the humeral component and to allow full extension

- A trial humeral component is then placed to verify the humeral cut height and quality of preparation of the humeral canal

Ulnar preparation

- Resection of tip of the olecranon is performed
- A high-speed burr is angled at 45° relative to the axis of the ulnar shaft at the junction of the sigmoid fossa and coronoid to identify the ulnar medullary canal
- A twist reamer is then used to further identify the canal, and progressively sized ulnar rasps are inserted
- The dorsal ulnar cortex is palpated while inserting the rasp to avoid ulnar perforation. The handle of the rasp must stay perpendicular to the flat, dorsal aspect of the olecranon. Small reamers can also be used on a guide wire is the canal is very small
- A trial ulnar component is then inserted to a depth such that the center of the ulnar component is midway between the tips of the olecranon and the coronoid to reproduce the elbow's axis of rotation
- A rongeur is the used to remove the tip of the coronoid to avoid impingement of the humeral component in flexion

Radial head

- Radial head resection is performed if degenerative lesions are identified. If intact, the radial head can be preserved

Trial reduction

- The humeral component is then inserted and the two components are coupled

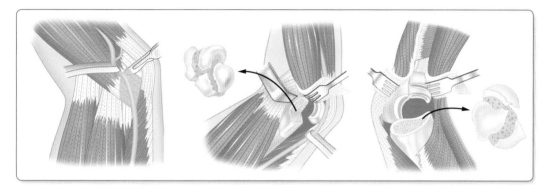

Figure 18.4 The triceps-sparing approach for a distal humeral fracture.

- Range of motion is tested in flexion and extension to confirm the full range of motion
- If the range of motion is limited, this can be due to bone impingement and/or inadequate soft tissue release

Cementing

- A cement restrictor is placed in both medullary canals, and pulse lavage is performed
- Low-viscosity cement with antibiotics is then injected using a special gun with a nozzle shortened to the length of the prosthesis.
- The nozzle presented with the gun is usually too long so it is shortened to the level of the stem used, i.e. 10 cm stem requires a 10 cm nozzle

Implant assembly

- After cement injection, the ulnar component is positioned first, and then the humeral component is engaged
- A bone graft harvested from the trochlea is positioned behind the anterior flange
- The components are then linked
- The humeral component is impacted (**Figure 18.5**)
- The elbow is then held in full extension while the cement hardens

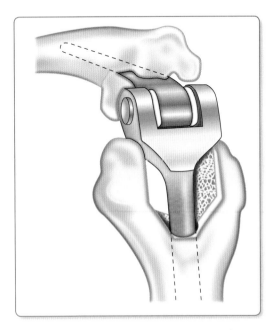

Figure 18.5 Assembly of the Coonrad–Morrey prosthesis.

Surgical technique for the convertible Latitude prosthesis (Tornier)

Humeral preparation

- Sizing of the patient's trochlea with the spool is critical. The spool must then be aligned to the trochlear groove of the ulna and the center of the radial head
- A cut is made at the center of the trochlea to allow access to the medullary canal
- A high-speed burr is used to open the medullary canal. A starting broach is then inserted until the flexion–extension line is aligned with the patient's flexion–extension axis
- Humeral broaching is performed sequentially to the select the humeral component size
- The trochlear cut guide is attached to the final broach. An oscillating saw is used to cut the trochlea around the guide
- The appropriate side, size, and length humeral stem trial with the corresponding humeral spool trial are placed in the humeral shaft

Ulnar preparation

- An ulnar jig is used with the sizing spool into the greater sigmoid notch of the ulna. The capitellar portion should align and articulate with the center of the radial head
- The post of the ulnar jig is slid into the sizing spool, and the clamp is tightened until the jig is secure on the flat portion of the olecranon
- A bell saw adapted to the size of the spool is used to cut the ulna. Ensure the ulnar nerve is protected when making this cut
- The radial head can be resected if needed with the same jig
- The ulnar canal is opened using a burr, and flexible reamers are used to further open the canal
- Ulnar broaching is then sequentially used parallel to the flat posterior portion of the proximal ulna
- The correct ulnar stem trial is impacted

Radial head preparation

- The trial radial head prosthesis adapted to the size of the ulnar component and humeral component is positioned in the radial canal

Trial reduction

- The elbow is reduced with the three components positioned

- The elbow should articulate through a full range of motion testing for stability, articular tracking, and axis of rotation
- If the trial reduction is not satisfactory, check that the trial implants are correctly positioned and that no soft tissue impingement has occurred. Check for impingement of the coronoid process on the anterior flange of the humeral component in flexion, and impingement of the olecranon process on the humeral component in extension, and resect as required
- In case of an unstable elbow, use the trial cap to link the implant
- If the trial radial head implant articulates congruently with the capitellum, a radial head component should be employed. However, if maltracking of the radial trial is evident, a radial head replacement should not be performed and the prosthesis must be linked

Linking the implant
- Because the Latitude prosthesis is a convertible implant, it can be used unlinked or linked
- To link the implant, an ulnar cap allows closing of the ulnar ring component around the humeral spool

Cementing
- The cementing technique is similar to that used for the Coonrad–Morrey prosthesis

Implants assembly
- After cement injection, the ulnar component is positioned first, and then the humeral component is engaged
- The radial head prosthesis if needed is also cemented
- A bone graft harvested from the trochlea is positioned behind the anterior flange
- The components are reduced
- If there is any instability or if the surgeon chooses, the implant is linked
- The elbow is then held in full extension while the cement hardens (**Figure 18.6**)

Triceps reinsertion
- Triceps reinsertion will depend on the triceps approach:
  - For a triceps-sparing approach, only the lateral and the medial windows are sutured
  - For a triceps-reflecting approach, three bone tunnels are made in the olecranon: two oblique and one transverse. A no. 5 nonabsorbable suture is then placed from distal to proximal into the distal medial oblique tunnel, and the suture is woven through the triceps tendon in a locking, crisscross pattern such that the suture emerges at the proximal medial hole. The suture is then passed through the other oblique tunnel. A transverse suture is passed through the triceps tendon from medial to lateral using the Mason-Allen technique. The sutures are then tied with the elbow flexed to 90°, beginning with the oblique sutures. Finally, the forearm aponeurosis is closed (**Figure 18.7**)

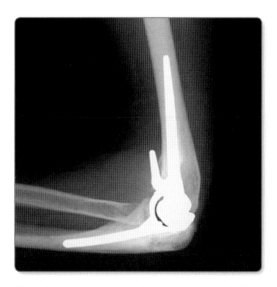

Figure 18.6 Radiograph showing the Latitude prosthesis.

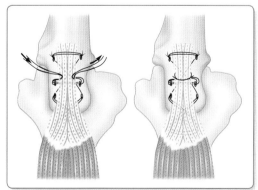

Figure 18.7 Repair following the triceps-reflecting approach.

- – The triceps-splitting approach should be carefully repaired using nonabsorbable locking Krachow sutures placed through drill holes in the ulna
- A cannulated humeral bolt in the humeral spool of the Latitude prosthesis allows the surgeon to repair the collateral ligaments as well as the common flexor and extensor origins to the implant

Ulnar nerve

- Depending on the position of the ulnar nerve at the end of the procedure, it can be left in place if there is no impingement of the prosthesis or any sign of instability
- If there is impingement or instability, the ulnar nerve is anteriorly transposed and stabilized in a subcutaneous pocket

Possible perioperative complications

Wound healing

- This is the most frequent complication
- The elbow joint is a superficial joint close to the subcutaneous tissue
- Patients with rheumatoid arthritis are often taking immunodepressant drugs that induce skin fragility
- In the context of trauma, the wound has been often injured by the trauma, hematoma, or previous surgeries
- For patients with fragile skin, adhesive dressings must be avoided
- The incision must be straight and lateralized to avoid overlying the olecranon tip. If previous incisions exist, they must be used again. If a new incision is chosen, a large enough intact skin bridge must be preserved between the two incisions
- Rigorous hemostasis must be performed after the tourniquet has been deflated to limit the risk of hematoma
- A drain is used for 24–48 hours
- The elbow is ideally immobilized for the first 2 days with an anterior splint to preserve the incision
- The wound must be monitored before allowing the patient to move the elbow
- Skin necrosis must be excised, and adapted coverage must be performed to protect the prosthesis

Perioperative fractures

- Column fractures are not uncommon during trochlear osteotomy. The cutting guide must be centered to avoid this complication
- With a linked prosthesis, an implant with an anterior flange must be inserted that improves stability
- With an unlinked prosthesis, reconstruction of the columns must be performed to enhance stability
- For periprosthetic fractures, a cerclage wire is usually used to stabilize the bone around the prosthesis, and a long-stem prosthesis is used that bypasses the fracture

Ulnar nerve compromise

- Ulnar nerve dysfuction after total elbow arthroplasty can be due to various causes including excessive traction, perineural or epineural hematoma, mechanical compression during surgery, thermal necrosis from cement, devascularization by extensive release, and/or compression by excessive edema or a tight dressing
- Ulnar nerve neurolysis is essential to avoid excessive traction during total elbow arthroplasty
- Manipulation of the nerve must be gentle during surgery. At the end of the procedure, the nerve is left alone or anteriorly transposed depending on the local condition

Triceps insufficiency

- Triceps insufficiency after a total elbow arthroplasty involves either a complete or partial rupture or avulsion of the triceps tendon from the olecranon
- It is perhaps the most infrequently recognized complication after total elbow arthroplasty. The reason for this is that patients can extend their elbow by using gravity and therefore unless it is specifically looked for it is easily missed. It is only with the arm elevated that weakness of extension becomes obvious
- It is more likely to occur in patients who have had previous surgery but is also influenced by the surgical approach. It has been shown to be mostly related to an inverted-V triceps approach compared to a triceps-reflecting approach or triceps-splitting approach
- A rigorous repair and postoperative protection allow satisfactory triceps healing. Triceps lengthening must be avoided

Infection

- Infection is the most devastating complication after total elbow arthroplasty
- The infection rate has been reported to be around 5% and can be decreased by adequate preoperative evaluation to rule out any infection, stopping immunodepressant drugs if possible, prescribing antibiotic prophylaxis, using cement with antibiotics, and rigorously monitoring wound healing

Instability

- This is the most frequent complication observed with an unlinked prosthesis
- It can be avoided by a rigorous selection of patients, attention to the choice of the type of implant, adequate positioning of the components, and a good balancing of the soft tissues around the joint
- Postoperative immobilization for 3–6 weeks in slight flexion can be useful before starting motion

Closure

- Wounds are closed in layers, and a drain is placed for 2 days

Postoperative management

- A volar splint is placed with the elbow in full extension for 2 days before the splint and drain are removed
- If a linked prosthesis is used, the patient is then allowed to actively flex the elbow, and passively extend it. No physical therapy is usually necessary
- If an unlinked prosthesis has been used, the elbow is immobilized at 60° in a well-padded splint for 15 days depending on the skin quality
- 15 days postoperatively, action flexion and gravity-assisted extension are performed with the forearm in neutral rotation
- Active extension is avoided for 6 weeks to protect the triceps repair

Outpatient follow-up

Patients have regular check ups:

- At 3 weeks to control wound healing and remove stitches
- At 3 months to control motion recovery and to make a radiographic analysis
- At 1 year for clinical and radiographic evaluation
- And then each year following

Further reading

Elhassan B, Ramsey ML, Steinmann SP. Management of primary degenerative arthritis of the elbow: linkable total elbow replacement. In: Wiesel SW (ed.), Operative techniques in orthopaedic surgery. Philadelphia: Wolters Kluwer, Lippincott Williams & Wilkins, 2010:3444–3452.

King GJW. Convertible total elbow arthroplasty. In: Morrey BF (ed.), The elbow and its disorders, 4th edn. Philadelphia: Saunders Elsevier, 2009.

Loeffler BJ, Connor PM. Total elbow arthroplasty for rheumatoid arthritis. In: Wiesel SW (ed.), Operative techniques in orthopaedic surgery. Philadelphia: Wolters Kluwer, Lippincott Williams & Wilkins, 2010: 3420–3432.

Morrey BF. Linked elbow arthroplasty: rationale, indications, and surgical technique. In: Morrey BF (ed.), The elbow and its disorders, 4th edn. Philadelphia: Saunders Elsevier, 2009.

Endoscopic treatment of olecranon bursitis

Indications

Endoscopic treatment of olecranon bursitis is indicated in:

- Patients with sterile oleranon bursitis unresponsive to nonoperative treatments such as rest, ice, anti-inflammatory drugs, aspiration, steroid injections, and compressive bandages
- Patients with treated infected olecranon bursitis undergoing excision of bursal tissue to prevent further infections

Preoperative assessment

Clinical assessment

Basic signs of olecranon bursitis

- Patients describe persistent swelling and pain over the tip of the elbow
- There is a limited range of motion in the elbow

Further physical assessment

- Assess the presence of swelling, tenderness, and erythema
- Assess the presence and degree of limitation of the range of motion
- Evaluate the presence of rheumatologic conditions associated with olecranon bursitis, and inform patients about the possibility of higher recurrence and complication rates following surgery

Imaging assessment

Radiographs

- Anteroposterior and lateral radiographs are performed to exclude possible olecranon fractures, and to detect arthritis and bone spurs on the olecranon tip

Ultrasonography

- Ultrasonography may be helpful in detecting effusions, synovial hypertrophy, calcifications, and loose bodies

Magnetic resonance imaging (MRI)

- When symptoms are severe, MRI helps to identify abscesses and osteomyelitis, and to differentiate septic bursitis from aseptic bursitis

Timing for surgery

- In sterile olecranon bursitis resistant to nonoperative treatment
- Patients with treated infected olecranon bursitis undergoing excision of bursal tissue to prevent further infections
- When there is a thickened bursal wall with fibrinous loose bodies, which is usually unresponsive to nonoperative treatment

Surgical preparation

Surgical equipment

The arthroscopic set includes a 4 mm 30° angled arthroscope and Karl Storz endoscopic instrument set including:

- A 3.5 mm resector
- A 3.5 mm burr
- Grasping forceps
- A probe

Equipment positioning

- The arthroscopic tower faces the surgeon on the opposite side of the table

Patient positioning

- The patient is placed in the lateral decubitus position with the involved extremity facing upward. The arm is stabilized on a padded bolster (arm holder) with the shoulder abducted to 90° and the elbow flexed to 90° (**Figure 19.1**)
- A tourniquet is applied to the upper arm
- Ensure that the patient's spine and pressure points of the arms and legs are protected by padding after final positioning

Further preparation

- Prophylactic antibiotics are given 30 minutes before surgery according to local hospital policy and guidelines
- The arm is prepared with an antiseptic solution to ensure sterility

Surgical technique

- Inflate the tourniquet to 250 mmHg
- With a sterile surgical skin pen, mark the bursal sac and ulnar nerve
- Distention of the bursa with an injection of saline helps its identification
- Make a 1–2 cm incision lateral to the bursal sac margin at the proximal aspect of the bursa (**Figure 19.2**)
- To create a working space, elevate the subcutaneous fat off the olecranon and bursal sac with forceps

- Using blunt dissection and under direct vision, insert the endoscope subcutaneously. Use low pressure to prevent overdistention
- Make a 1–2 cm incision medial to the bursal sac margin at the proximal aspect of the bursa (**Figure 19.2**)
- Elevate the subcutaneous fat and connect the portals by creating a space between the subcutaneous fat and bursal sac
- Resect the fibrous bands, synovial tissue, and thickened bursal sac with a resector
- Ensure complete resection of the bursal tissue until the fibers of the triceps tendon are seen; care is taken not to perforate the skin and not to damage the ulnar nerve
- Remove any bone spurs on the olecranon tip by using a burr
- Deflate the tourniquet
- Ensure there is no bleeding in the resected area that can cause a hematoma

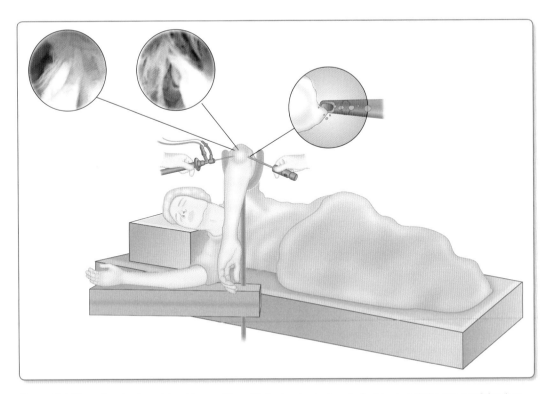

Figure 19.1 The patient in a lateral decubitus position with the involved extremity facing upward. The arm is stabilized on a padded bolster (arm holder) with the shoulder abducted to 90° and the elbow flexed to 90°. Fibrous bands and synovial hypertrophy are seen and the bursal sac is resected using an endoscopic technique.

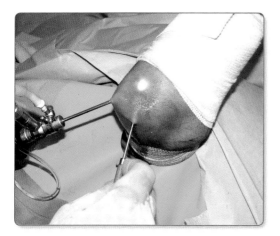

Figure 19.2 The lateral portal is located 1–2 cm lateral to the bursal sac margin on the proximal aspect of the bursa. The medial portal is located 1–2 cm medial to the the bursal sac margin on the proximal aspect of the bursa.

Possible perioperative complications

- Skin perforation when performing blunt dissection. This will need to be repaired and a compressive dressing applied
- Ulnar nerve injury

Closure

- Close the skin with monofilament sutures
- Apply a compressive dressing

Postoperative management

Postoperative regimen

- Medications: analgesia and nonsteroidal anti-inflammatory drugs
- Gentle active range of motion exercises are allowed postoperatively
- Patients are seen after 1 week for wound review and dressing
- Advise patients to avoid heavy activities and excessive pressure over the olecranon for 6 weeks

Early-phase postoperative complications

- Hematoma formation. Prevention involves hemostasis after tourniquet deflation and compressive bandages
- Formation of a persistent sinus from skin perforation

Further reading

Blankstein A, Ganel A, Givon U, et al. Ultrasonographic findings in patients with olecranon bursitis. Ultraschall Med 2006; 27:568–571.

Kerr DR, Carpenter CW. Arthroscopic resection of olecranon and prepatellar bursae. Arthroscopy 1990; 6:86–88.

Ogilvie-Harris DJ, Gilbart M. Endoscopic bursal resection: the olecranon bursa and prepatellar bursa. Arthroscopy 2000; 16:249–253.